"This book will resonate with countless people who have experienced the beauty and pain of walking beside someone they love through illness. Wonderfully written and perfectly titled, this book makes me want to be a better doctor and a better husband."

–Dr. Cameron McLaren
Medical Oncologist and Founder, Voluntary Assisted Dying Australia and New Zealand (VADANZ)

"Stephanie Duran addresses a critical and emotionally laden topic in a clear-eyed, heartfelt love letter to her husband, friend, lover, and soulmate. It is written in the first person, so personal, by an author willing and able to be vulnerable. It also tells in searing detail the journey of two lovers willing to be courageous enough to describe dying with dignity. I am sure this will speak to not only those who experienced the same wrenching feelings and actions, but to those who may be considering dying with dignity."

–Dr. Richard Boxer, MD, FACS
Professor at UCLA, Twice Presidential Appointee to the National Cancer Advisory Board

"Stephanie Duran's book is a very moving and important one for the public to read about, and it is also a wonderful love story."

–Dame Janet Suzman
Academy Award Oscar Nominee for Best Actress

"Beautifully-written and a must read for patients and their family members who have to navigate through cancer."

–Dr. Arya Amini, MD
Associate Professor, Department of Radiation Oncology

"Love can be all consuming and bring great joy to those lucky enough to experience it. Stephanie Duran was one of the lucky ones. However, we never know what challenges tomorrow will bring. This exceptionally well-written book is a true story of great love impacted by a journey through unbelievable pain and suffering. It is both heartwarming and heart-wrenching as this partnership deals with life's lottery."

–**Dr. Tom McKaskill**
Author, Ph.D, CPA

"This is not a book about cancer, though it is. Nor is it a love story, although you will fall in love with Stephanie and Jeff. Neither is it a commentary on values, but it will challenge you and open your mind. Ultimately, this is a book about all of us… and an invitation to rise to life!"

–**Dan Gregory**
Author, Award-Winning Thought Leader, and Keynote Speaker

Surviving The Unthinkable

BECAUSE I LOVED YOU

A Memoir
STEPHANIE DURAN

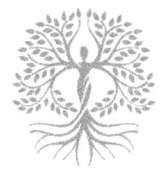

JT PUBLISHING HOUSE
Because I Loved You
Copyright © 2025 Stephanie Duran
Names: Duran, Stephanie.
Title: Because/ Stephanie Duran.

Summary: "Because I Loved You is a breathtaking memoir that begins as a once-in-a-lifetime love story and transforms into a courageous, heart-wrenching journey through terminal illness and the powerful, legal choice to die with dignity in California."— Provided by the author.

Identifiers: ISBN 979-8-9998160-0-9 (paperback)
ISBN 979-8-9998160-1-6 (hardback)
ISBN 979-8-9998160-2-3 (ebook)

Subjects: BISAC: SELF-HELP / Death, Grief, Bereavement
BIOGRAPHY & AUTOBIOGRAPHY / Personal Memoirs

Library of Congress Control Number: 2025945871

This Revised Edition reflects updates and improvements made since the original publication. While the heart of the book remains the same, I've expanded and refined several sections, clarified ideas, added reflective journal prompts, and made updates to ensure the content continues to serve readers in the best way possible.

This book is a work of non-fiction. Unless otherwise noted, the author and the publisher make no explicit guarantees as to the accuracy of the information contained in this book and in some cases, names of people and places have been altered to protect their privacy.

Because of the dynamic nature of the Internet, any web addresses or links contained in this book may have changed since publication and may no longer be valid. The views expressed in this work are solely those of the author and do not necessarily reflect the views of the publisher, and the publisher hereby disclaims any responsibility for them.

The author of this book does not dispense medical advice or prescribe the use of any technique as a form of treatment for physical, emotional, or medical problems without the advice of a physician, either directly or indirectly. The intent of the author is only to offer information of a general nature to help you in your quest for emotional and spiritual well-being. In the event you use any of the information in this book for yourself, which is your constitutional right, the author and the publisher assume no responsibility for your actions.

All rights reserved. No part of this publication may be reproduced, stored in a retrieval system, or transmitted in any form or by any means—electronic, mechanical, photocopying, recording, or any other—except for brief quotations in printed reviews, without the prior permission of the publisher, as permitted under Section 107 or 108 of the 1976 United States Copyright Act, without either the prior written permission of the author or authorization through payment of the appropriate per-copy fee to the Copyright Clearance Center, Inc. 222 Rosewood Drive, Danvers, MA 01923, 978-750-8400, fax 978-646-8600, or on the web at www.copyright.com.

All rights reserved.

Published by JT Publishing, Spartanburg, South Carolina
www.jtpublishinghouse.com
Printed in the United States of America

10 9 8 7 6 5 4 3 2

TABLE OF CONTENTS

Dedication xi
Acknowledgments xiii
Book Reviews xv
Chapter 1 — Run 1
Chapter 2 — The Gamble..9
Chapter 3 — Surf And Sand 19
Chapter 4 — Together 27
Chapter 5 — New Beginnings 39
Chapter 6 — Just Breathe 47
Chapter 7 — Desperate Measures 57
Chapter 8 — Summer After The Diagnosis...............................71
Chapter 9 — The Plan 81
Chapter 10 — Summer Of Hell...91
Chapter 11 — Recovery 99
Chapter 12 — Rearrange 111
Chapter 13 — Delirious 121
Chapter 14 — Unforgettable 129
Chapter 15 — Spiraling 139
Chapter 16 — Stretched Thin 153
Chapter 17 — Backyard Secrets...161
Chapter 18 — The Final Ring 171
Chapter 19 — Four Words 189
Chapter 20 — Toodle-oo 199
Chapter 21 — Ashes...215
Chapter 22 — A Second Sunrise 229
Epilogue...245

DEDICATION

There were four conversations I needed to have before I could begin writing this memoir:

This book is for the love I had to say goodbye to, the love I opened my heart to once again, and my two extraordinary children, who have walked every step of this journey beside me.

To my love, **Jeff Dunphy**—

You breathed life into a heart that didn't even know it was waiting for you. I never knew love could feel the way it did until I met you. Your compassionate, courageous soul wanted our story shared, reminding me so often, "If our story could help even just one, then Honeybee, you need to tell it." Your bravery, your fight for time, your boundless love—they gifted us more memories than I could have ever dreamed. I am eternally grateful. Your legacy of kindness, strength, and love will live on, touching hearts long after these pages are turned. My heart finds you every single day—and it always will.

To my new love, **Tim Sturm**—

Thank you for the extraordinary grace and generosity you have shown, not only to me but to my children. You embrace all the pieces of my story, honoring the man you never knew with a tenderness and selflessness that are rare and breathtaking. Your patient heart and unwavering support—through every late night of writing, every tear, and every memory—have made it possible for me to honor the past while building something beautiful and new with you. Loving you feels like a second sunrise, a blessing I never take for granted.

To my children, **Maddie and Jake**—

There are no words strong enough to hold the gratitude, pride, and pure love I feel for you both. Watching you open your hearts first to Jeff, creating bonds that enriched all our lives, and then courageously embracing Tim with the same warmth and authenticity, is the greatest testament to the incredible souls you are. Your capacity to love, to trust, to build, and to welcome joy again humbles me daily. Being your mama will forever be the greatest and purest joy of my life.

This book is dedicated to and in honor of all those who have walked this path, and to those just beginning:

Never let a diagnosis dictate your destiny.

ACKNOWLEDGMENTS

Each time I cross a finish line, I make it a point to slow down, breathe deeply, reflect, and honor every step that carried me there.

On my fifty-fifth birthday, August 17, 2023, sitting beneath a sun-drenched sky on the patio of a winery, surrounded by dear friends, laughter, and glasses raised in celebration, I made a quiet, powerful declaration to them. I drew in a steady breath and released the words I had cradled in my heart for over three years: "I'm going to write a book. I'm going to be an author." Speaking it aloud made it real; there would be no turning back. It wasn't just my journey—it was ours. As their cheers and love wrapped around me, my heart swelled with gratitude. And just like that, in March 2024, a new chapter of my life began.

At the very start of this journey, New York Times best-selling author Don Bentley generously gifted me his time and wisdom. On January 1, 2024, he walked through my vision and concept with me, offering invaluable advice that propelled me into the world of authorship. His encouragement lit the first spark that would grow into this book.

I am deeply grateful to my writing coaches and editors, Michelle Black and Scott Huesing, whose insight and steady guidance shaped the soul of this manuscript. To Michelle—my editor and weekly partner through every twist and turn—you helped me find and trust my writer's voice. You encouraged me to step beyond my comfort zone to bring the story of Jeff and me to life with honesty and heart. Your unwavering support, patience, and belief in this story made all the difference. I will always carry deep gratitude for you both.

To my daughter, Maddie Elie—thank you for bravely taking on the first round of edits. It was an emotional labor of love, and having you help shape this story was one of the greatest gifts of all. To Ethan Raye, my gifted copy editor, thank you for putting the final polish on every page with care and precision.

To Monica Kline and the Identity Brand team—thank you for helping to bring my vision to life and build something far beyond a book. From a single, heartfelt idea, you helped me build more than a brand; you helped me shape a mission to guide professionals in supporting others through life's most profound losses and transitions.

We offer our heartfelt and deepest gratitude to the extraordinary teams at City of Hope, Loma Linda Hospital, UCLA Hospital, and Tufts Medical Center. Your kindness, patience, and unwavering commitment gifted us something priceless—more time. Your efforts gave Jeff and me the hope and strength we needed to endure some of the hardest moments of our journey. There are no words big enough to hold our gratitude.

I would also like to extend my heartfelt thanks to my photographers. Thank you to Alex Nguyen of Février Photography, in Paris, France, for beautifully capturing our love story on our 2019 Paris trip, portrayed on the front cover. And a special thank you to Tony Lattimore Photography, in Orange County, CA, for warmly capturing my author bio photo on the back cover.

I also want to recognize JT Publishing House, for bringing this labor of love to life with such care.

To my children, my parents, my new love, all our loving family and friends across the U.S., Canada, the U.K., and Australia—you were our lifeline. You lifted Jeff and me during the darkest hours after his diagnosis, held me through my healing, and stood by me every step of this writing journey. Your encouragement, prayers, and unwavering love have been an indescribable blessing.

Finally, to Jeff—

Your love, courage, selflessness, and extraordinary bravery are woven into every word of this story. Your love shaped my journey then and continues to inspire every breath of my future.

BOOK REVIEWS

"Stephanie's deeply moving memoir touched my heart in unexpected ways. It's a powerful personal story of love, loss, and learning how to love again after unimaginable pain. It brings hope and strength to anyone caring for a loved one with a long-term illness and sparks inspiration to live life fully present, seizing the ordinary, everyday moments as the most precious. Thank you for helping us all to embrace the now and to see the light in life's darkest times."

–Jenni Simmons

"*Because I Loved You* is one of the most moving books I've ever read. Stephanie's writing drew me in immediately–beautiful, heartfelt, and so real that I found myself turning page after page, unable to stop. Her story about her relationship with Jeff and their journey after his terminal cancer diagnosis is deeply personal yet filled with universal life lessons that anyone can take to heart. This book made me cry, but it also lifted me with moments of love and joy. It touched my soul in a way few books ever have, and I'll carry its message with me for a long time."

–Jill Klinge

"Stephanie and Jeff's journey is both beautiful and heartbreaking. Hopefully, sharing it will help others not only cope with their grief but also continue to live. This story shows us all that it's not easy, but with love and support, it's possible to keep living and loving while missing and grieving for a lost love."

–Ellen S.

"The love story of Stephanie and Jeff was absolutely beautiful. We all say the vows "in sickness and in health," but Stephanie and Jeff lived them. While their relationship was so inspiring, it's Stephanie's ability to jump in with both feet and fully commit to an adventure or love without knowing the outcome that I found inspiring. It has made me realize that we should all strive to live that way because that's how you find magic."

–**Christine Horowitz**

"What a story of hope and healing. Stephanie inspires others that there's love after loss and that no matter your heartache, you can come out the other side. Inspiring, uplifting, and helpful to anyone dealing with loss or grieving. Highly recommend this read!"

–**Heather Torigian**

"In her book, *Because I Loved You*," Stephanie shares her journey of love & loss. The tone of her story is raw and authentic, allowing readers to really connect with what she went through. Her voice is tender and caring yet strong & powerful. So many people will benefit from reading this book."

–**Jacki Riggs**

"This book didn't just move me, it changed my perspective on life and how to live it. It showed me how to find joy even in the darkest moments. Reading this story taught me to treat hardships not as burdens but as lessons and beautiful challenges to overcome."

–**Jacob Elie**

"This book has touched my heart. The love, the courage, and the promises between two people were so powerful and inspiring. Jeff and Stephanie both loved with all of their hearts. He wanted her to share their story to help at least one person, and it will help so many more. The way that Stephanie was able to pick herself up through the grief and move on was so inspiring. She was so brave and found new love. Thank you for sharing your story. It gives hope to so many others."

–**Margo McGee**

"Wow! From the first page to the last, I was engaged in the whole story; love and compassion fly off the pages. What a powerful way to honor the love of your life! Compassion, raw emotion, and honesty. Stephanie writes with care and humility, opening her heart so others may see hope as they face their greatest loss."

–**Michelle E.**

"*Because I Loved You* is a heartfelt journey that touched my heart with both tears and smiles. The love story between Stephanie and Jeff, though tragically cut short, shines brightly through these pages. Stephanie endured the unimaginable loss of her love. Now she uses her experiences to bless and help others after the loss of a loved one. She's turned something good out of the tragedy, and that's the example we all need to remember: no matter what losses we face, through resilience, we can persevere."

–**Janet F.**

"Stephanie's book deeply moved me. Her vulnerability in sharing the pain of losing her true love, Jeff, and the healing journey that followed, is both powerful and inspiring. The way she turns personal grief into a message of hope and healing is a true testament to her strength. Her story is a gift to anyone navigating loss, a reminder that even in heartbreak, love endures and purpose can rise from pain."

–**Kimberly Wright**

"While reading this book, I felt every emotion imaginable. I laughed, I cried, I smiled, and I felt the strength of their true love pouring out of every page. I would highly recommend this book to anyone experiencing a great loss."

–**Maddie Elie**

"I felt the strength, hope, and courage of two people in love. What touched me the most was one of the last paragraphs, which highlighted that most things in life are temporary and that obstacles in our path are opportunities for growth. That seemed to sum up this beautiful yet heartbreaking story."

–**Stephanie Anastos-Ratner**

"*Because I Loved You*, by Stephanie Duran, reached the depths of my heart and soul. The loss of a loved one is part of life that many people go through, but rarely speak of after the initial pain and sorrow. This memoir allows its readers to go on a spiritual and emotional journey. It beautifully describes both trials and triumphs that resonate with everyone who has ever felt a profound loss. More importantly, the author leaves you with a sense of hope, inspiration, and a true belief that love is never-ending and can be found again if you choose to seek joy."

–**Laura Gilden**

"A true labor of love, "*Because I Loved You*" is a memoir written with raw emotion and honest openness that takes readers on a very personal, heartfelt journey of love, loss, grief, and healing. It is an inspiring story that reminds us you're not alone and that you can "survive the unthinkable."

–**Timothy S.**

"After reading Stephanie Duran's book "*Because I loved You*," it really put life, love, and companionship into perspective. Time and love are not a given, so when true love is found, we must learn to cherish every moment we have together. Thank you, Stephanie, for sharing your beautiful story. This will be an inspiration for all."

–**Vanessa Velez**

"After finishing the book, I found myself hugging my husband a little longer, reminded of the importance of not taking a single moment for granted. The story Stephanie shares is not only a testament to the power of love but also a reminder to live fully and fearlessly. It's an inspiring read that will touch your heart and motivate you to cherish every moment."

–**Kathryn Boulanger**

"*Because I Loved You* is more than a memoir; it's a lifeline for anyone who has ever suffered loss. Stephanie Duran writes with such honesty and vulnerability that you feel seen in your own grief, no matter what form it has taken. Her story shows that loss is not a single moment in time but a journey we walk every day, through love and pain, and ultimately toward healing. What makes this book so powerful is how it gently helps you understand that grief is not something to "get over," but something you learn to carry. Stephanie's courage in sharing her deepest heartbreak reminds us that even in the darkest moments, there is hope, meaning, and joy again. This book gave me comfort, perspective, and the reassurance that love never truly leaves us. For anyone navigating loss, whether it's the death of a partner, family member, friend, or any goodbye, *Because I Loved You* will speak to your heart and help you feel less alone."

–Adriana Brusi

This Book is a Resource for Professionals Supporting Clients through Loss and Transition

BECAUSE I LOVED YOU

A memoir that reveals the human side of financial planning, loss, and legacy.

When we received a terminal cancer diagnosis, life changed overnight. What followed was a journey through caregiving, difficult decisions, grief, and rebuilding, offering a rare firsthand perspective on what families truly experience during life's most challenging transitions.

Because I Loved You is more than a personal story. It is a powerful lens into the emotional realities that often sit behind financial conversations, helping professionals better understand the people they serve.

WHY THIS BOOK MATTERS

Financial planners and advisors are often present during some of life's most sensitive moments. This memoir offers insight into:

- The emotional weight clients carry into financial decisions
- How grief and stress impact timing, communication, and clarity
- The importance of empathy alongside expertise
- What families wish professionals understood during crisis and transition
- This book helps bridge the gap between strategy and humanity for professionals across medical, legal, financial, and all client-facing services

ABOUT STEPHANIE DURAN

Stephanie Duran is an author, speaker, attorney, and educator who helps financial professionals better understand the human experience behind wealth, legacy, and life transitions. Through lived experience and storytelling, she brings depth, perspective, and compassion to conversations that matter most.

Firms and advisors use Because I Loved You for:

- Client support and thoughtful gifting
- Advisor education and team development
- Legacy and estate planning conversations
- Professional development and empathy training

Behind every financial plan is a human story.

Because I Loved You invites professionals to lead with both expertise and understanding.

"Stephanie Duran's presentation was an incredibly touching and honest perspective that relates directly to the work we do with our clients during life's transitions. She reminded us that our clients will remember how we made them feel above all else and that being present and compassionate is essential."

–**Andre L.**
Sentinel Wealth Advisory Group, Ameriprise Financial Services

"Stephanie Duran delivered one of the most powerful and emotionally resonant presentations I've experienced at any professional event. Speaking as both a seasoned attorney and a widow who lost her husband to cancer, she offered a rare and compelling blend of professional expertise and deeply personal insight that moved every person in the room.

You could have heard a pin drop as she shared not only her personal story, but also actionable, compassionate strategies for supporting widowed clients with integrity, empathy, and presence. Her authenticity, strength, and clarity held our attention from the first moment to the last.

What she delivered wasn't just a talk; it was a masterclass in how to meet grieving clients in their most vulnerable moments and how to serve them in a way that builds lifelong trust. Stephanie's guidance was not only relevant, practical, and informative, it was transformative."

–**Jill Klinge**
Attorney

"Stephanie's keynote was unlike anything I've experienced in my 23-year career. In a profession that rarely pauses to address the human side of what we do, her talk hit me straight in the heart. Her story was deeply personal, but the way she connected it to how we show up for clients, especially those navigating grief or loss, was powerful and practical. I walked away with new language, a deeper sense of empathy, and a reminder that honoring humanity is not just compassionate, it's good business."

–**Timothy S.**
Financial Services

"After hearing Stephanie speak, it taught me that our small actions can have a meaningful impact on our clients and help build trust. Today also taught me that it's important to show our clients that we're walking alongside them during a painful time."

–**Iris L.**
Sentinel Wealth Advisory Group, Ameriprise Financial Services

"Stephanie brought a professional vulnerability to the event; it was a rare and unforgettable combination. She didn't just inspire; she equipped us with relevant tools. Stephanie's talk guided the high-performing professionals in the room on how to better understand and prepare for those unexpected moments. She left me wanting more."

–**Gill Carr**
Executive Producer, Moody Street Kids Pty Lt

I would love to stay connected. You can reach me at: stephanie@thestephanieduran.com

Visit me online:

Follow me on Instagram:

Chapter 1
RUN

The light was low in the sky as I stepped out my front door, shutting it gingerly behind me. It was clear the marine layer would burn off early, and it would be another beautiful, hot September day in Southern California. Snuggly lacing up my old Asics running shoes, I set out for my daily run along the rolling, tree-lined hills through the neighborhood where I had lived for twenty-five years. As I allowed my body to warm up, my lungs breathed in the fragrance of blooming jasmine.

Over the past several years, I ran at every opportunity; it brought a sense of peace and solace. Private moments on the hot pavement were my solitude and time for reflection, allowing me to find my inner strength that was depleted every twenty-four hours. Running renewed me and gave me the ability to tackle the endless challenges that were brought into the beautiful life my fiancé, Jeff, and I had created. The minutes and miles I ran religiously every week refocused my thoughts as I ran through the pain, listening to my playlist, which I had purposefully called "Inspire."

I was acutely aware that daily moments of inspiration would help me find the strength I needed to fight another day. For me, private time alone, running, and meditating on God were necessary to face the insurmountable challenges ahead. Running was my lifeline, allowing me to return home feeling I could take on anything the day would throw at us. I felt strong after every run as the endorphins coursed through my body, filling my soul with hope, faith, and a chance to reconnect with God. My mind often wandered, recounting the endless, beautiful memories I shared with Jeff—traveling, filling our home with laughter, two-stepping at every opportunity, and touching each other as our hearts connected all day, every day since we first met.

When his gaze met mine years earlier, we could have never imagined that a chance encounter in our swimsuits and pool hats would blossom into a love story. At first glance, it would appear we lived polar opposite lifestyles. We soon discovered that we possessed so much more in common than we could imagine, all from a happenstance in an unlikely place far from home.

On that run, the morning of September 1, 2021, I couldn't help but think of the beautiful bouquet of my favorite flowers Jeff had sent me the day before. Knowing how much excruciating pain he was in made the gesture extraordinary, and I was in awe of how he could have found the energy to be so incredibly thoughtful. My heart was continually filled with love, appreciation, and gratitude for being gifted with such a remarkable soul to love.

Jeff put me first throughout our relationship; his adoration seemed effortless. He made sure that I always felt his loving heart wrapped around me every week, month, and year since our eyes first met. Every day, he found creative ways to ensure I knew how much he adored me. He left hundreds of love notes in my purse, on the bathroom mirror, in my car, in a drawer, and even in my sunglasses case. Many times, over the years, when I was out with girlfriends or family, he would call the restaurant to send over my favorite glass of wine or dessert for the table, attaching a sweet love note in the waitress's writing. The note always started with "Honeybee" and ended with "Love Always and Forever, Jeff." I never doubted his love for one second. It was unshakable. Neither the thousands of miles we lived apart for years, nor the horrific challenges we endured throughout our relationship, could alter our love for each other.

That day, as I ran along the path feeling safe while breathing in the jasmine and meditating on my love for Jeff, I could have never imagined what was in store for me when I returned home from my morning run.

I turned the knob and gently pushed open the green front door to our home, still panting heavily from the heat and miles I had just taken on. I set down my headphones, phone, and water bottle and headed upstairs to our bedroom to check on Jeff. I felt charged and ready for the day as I swiftly ascended the stairs two at a time, excited to kiss my love good morning.

What came next, I should have mentally prepared myself for better, but I hadn't; I'm not sure anyone can. I strolled into our bedroom and saw Jeff sitting quietly in the big, white, cozy corner chair. The armrests and back were slightly swayed after years of prolonged use, and the black floral swirl pattern had faded in the strong sunlight that poured through the bedroom windows each day. Jeff regularly sat by the picture window, watching the world outside and occasionally napping. The room felt quiet and peaceful. Seeing he was resting, I thought I would quietly sneak by to take a shower before starting our day. I turned my head to look back at him before heading into the bathroom, and our eyes met. I smiled at him with sweat streaming down my face and walked over to kiss him good morning. Leaning in, our lips gently touched, and our eyes locked.

Holding my gaze, Jeff took his long index finger and placed it over the tracheotomy to cover up the hole where air escaped; then he softly whispered four powerful words, his voice cracking and shaky. He wanted to ensure I didn't ask him to repeat himself as he looked up at me. "Today is the day."

Everything stopped. The room was like a vacuum; nothing moved. There was no air, the sound of blood rushing through my head was deafening, and I couldn't breathe. I knew what he meant, but I wanted to ask anyway. I needed to know for certain if he really meant what my mind wouldn't allow me to process. My inner voice told me, *No, it's not possible*. My heart knew, but my mind was still trying to comprehend; it just couldn't catch up. I could feel that pit in my throat, the one we get when our emotions are overwhelmed and the pain is trying to find its way out. Deep down, I knew what he meant, and I couldn't possibly ask him to repeat those words. I could only imagine the strength and courage it took for him to speak them once.

I could hear everything now, especially the clock. The seconds were so heavy that I could feel each one racing past me. *God, help me slow it down. Please stop time*, I thought, as a fear and panic I've never experienced began to set in. My mind turned to a place of comfort where I could allow myself to breathe.

I thought about the tiny, seemingly ordinary details of Jeff's life that I had the privilege of learning over the years. To me, Jeff was a bit of a walking contradiction. Raised in a small hamlet in the country with a population of eighty, he loved fine food, wine, worldly travel, and shopping. Things I would not naturally equate with my "farmer boy," a nickname I quickly gave him.

Jeff could fix anything. His upbringing led to his natural instinct to repair whatever he was confronted with: a car, a home, the yard, electrical, mechanical, or anything at all. Jeff always said, "If I can do it with my two hands, then I'm not going to pay someone else to repair it for me." Even if it was something he had never seen, it didn't matter. He would google it and ask anyone with expertise on the subject, and then somehow, with exact precision, he figured it out like a pro. His patience was unparalleled. He could spend hours tinkering and learning until he got it just right, rarely getting frustrated or angry in the process, regardless of how long it took; he had the patience of Job. He carried an obvious satisfaction throughout his entire being; when he successfully completed a project, he would glow like a child who had just received their first straight-A report card. Then he would open the fridge, proudly grab a well-deserved cold beer, and sit on the back patio, basking in the sun by the glistening pool, playing his favorite country tunes, and enjoying his well-earned afternoon on a perfect day. I fell so in love with his eagerness and ability to willingly take on any task.

His patience was reflected in many aspects of his life. From the everyday things like how he made his mouthwatering barbecue to how he would stand at the stove cooking bacon perfectly crispy for our Sunday brunches, while I made homemade waffles with fresh berries and cream. Although his patience was a prominent strength, it would run thin at times, and his temper would come barreling out. Everyone knew when he was about to lose his cool and did not want to be in his path when that temper swept through.

Jeff had a thirst for adventure, another love we shared. He loved to tell everyone the story of his backpacking and biking in the Canadian mountains in his younger days. On one trip, he was coming down a hill, unable to stop in time, went over a cliff, and landed on a small glacier. He was fearless—and fearless of rules at times. When we went out on a date, if I told him I loved the cute spoon or dish on the table at the restaurant, it would "somehow" end up in our home. I would jokingly say he was a bit of a "klepto." He lovingly took a few items over the years that didn't have a price tag. We had a collection from the places we patronized, and to this day, I see those items in the kitchen cabinet, and a smile stretches across my face.

We loved playing sports together. On one of our first trips to Palm Desert, he grabbed a football and tossed it to me, asking me to throw it around the pool. I motioned like Babe Ruth, pointing for him to go long, and I threw a spiral at his chest. You would have thought I threw the winning Super Bowl pass the way he cheered and hollered; we laughed hysterically and played in the pool all day. Skiing and golfing were some of the sports we enjoyed doing together in the winters in Canada and the springs in California.

Jeff was a walking Hallmark card. He knew exactly what to say to everyone he encountered. He was always on point for the occasion, whether it was humorous sarcasm or a beautiful compliment. He opened and held doors for everyone and was the first to jump in when he could see anyone, even a stranger, needing assistance. One time, he saved a woman's life at the racetrack in Edmonton, Canada. We had just come out of the bathroom when we heard a loud thud on the floor. Jeff knew immediately that someone had fallen; he said he could tell by the sound. He quickly jumped in, went to the woman's side, and started CPR. When she came to, he gently talked her through what had happened. As he spoke with her, he asked me to hold her hand while we waited for the paramedics.

His presence was humble and unassuming, yet he was never afraid. He would always get out on the dance floor with me and dance until sweat was dripping off us. He'd dance all night long with a cocktail in one hand and his other hand high in the air, fingers outstretched, pumping to the beat of the music. Never in a hurry, even on the LA freeways, letting everyone in if they wanted to change lanes; anyone from Southern California knows that's a rare sighting. He was a true gentleman. He had his flaws and imperfections, yet he was everything I needed.

Jeff's acute focus, patience, sense of humor, humility, and attention to detail guided his twenty-eight-year career as a respiratory therapist in the ICU at the Royal Alexandra Hospital (locals referred to it as "The Alec") in Edmonton. He was incredibly skilled and highly regarded in his field at The Alec. He cared for his patients and their families with the utmost attention, bringing them comfort and peace during difficult times. He had an innate ability to make the patient feel special, as though he had nothing but time and their best interests at heart. Jeff's extraordinary patience brought comfort and reassurance to his patients and their families when they feared for their loved one's serious respiratory condition, which often required a tracheotomy. Jeff rarely spoke in detail about his work, primarily because it had been mentally and emotionally exhausting working in the ICU for almost three decades. He occasionally shared some of the notes or kind words his patients and their families conveyed to him, expressing their heartfelt gratitude. They thanked him for treating them with such gentle care and thoughtfulness as if the patient were his own loved one.

Jeff had never been one to brag about his successes—how many lives he'd positively impacted or saved on his shifts—and he rarely discussed the painful losses. However, the thousands of lives he had directly affected were among his greatest gifts and contributions to the families he'd worked with in Canada.

Standing by his faded, white chair that September morning, the sweat dripping off my face turned cold as I worked to process the words Jeff had just spoken. The kind, caring, and gentle man who held my whole heart and had committed his to mine asked the unfathomable. Jeff had spent his career saving lives, but today, he asked me to help him take one. Today was the day we both dreaded and had fought so hard to avoid.

Today was the day Jeff decided he would die.

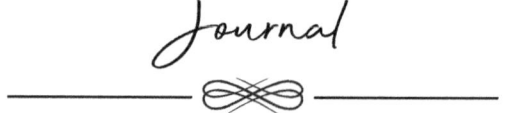

You've just walked with me through a morning that began with peace and ended with life-altering words. Sometimes in life, there are moments where the ordinary and the unthinkable collide. When you think about the rituals or practices that keep you steady in the storms of life, what comes to mind? Write about the ways you've found to hold on to your strength when the world shifts beneath your feet.

Chapter 2

THE GAMBLE

It was May 2014 when I left my home in Los Angeles, California, and boarded a flight to Las Vegas. I needed a lighthearted girls' weekend following my divorce. After a twenty-one-year marriage, I was feeling both crushed and uncertain of who I was as an individual. For so many years, I had been an "us," but suddenly, it was just me. I needed to get to know myself again.

I could smell the scent of orange blossoms and jasmine filling the warm, moist summer air as I made my way to catch the Vegas-bound flight out of Ontario, California. Anticipation of freedom and the festivities planned for our girls' trip filled my senses as we set out for my friend Heather's birthday celebration weekend. I had been to Vegas dozens of times over the years. The prior visits were the usual experience: gambling stories of how we hit it big or lost it all, and drinking stories that made you laugh until you cried. There were always memorable meals, celebrity shows, walking down the strip, people-watching, days at the pools, lots of laughter, and a unique feeling of playfulness that only Vegas can provide.

However, the memories from that trip would be unlike any other. A more perfect script could not have been written. That Vegas story would become one for the books. Wheels down, and that weekend began.

Knowing Vegas can be a pitfall for people coming out of a lonely place, I begrudgingly asked the birthday girl not to let me do anything stupid in Vegas. I knew I was vulnerable; I was in an unfamiliar place emotionally and wanted a second set of eyes to hold me accountable. We were in Sin City, after all, and shit happens more easily there. Being the great friend that she is, she took my request to heart, even on her birthday getaway.

The stars had aligned, though we couldn't see it. The first few days in Vegas were filled with the usual drinking, dancing, gambling, and endless laughter as we enjoyed our girl time. The new sense of freedom I felt that weekend was electrifying and rejuvenating.

We spent our last day in Vegas enjoying the pool. I've always loved meeting new people, hearing their stories, and learning the details of where they're from, so I walked around alone in the pool, making friends of all ages from around the world.

After a couple of hours of socializing in the pool with my cocktail in hand, I felt relaxed. The warm water lapped at my waist as the sun bronzed my shoulders and chest. For the first time in twenty years, I felt free and light. The weight of a thousand lifetimes had been lifted from me, and I glided along, blissfully sipping my vodka soda. I was a strong, independent woman with the whole world at my fingertips and a beautiful lifetime ahead of me filled with unknown opportunities. I smiled as I turned a corner and saw a man sitting on the pool's edge without a care in the world.

He was soaking in every ray of sunshine available that day. His hat was on backward, and he wore reflective Oakley sunglasses and a gold chain. A bucket of beers rested next to him. Something about his unassuming and handsome demeanor reminded me of Bradley Cooper. He sat on the edge of the pool, relaxing to the tunes that played over the loudspeakers as he tanned his shirtless, long, and lean body. He was hot.

At that moment, something came over me; maybe it was the cocktail, the freedom of my last day in Vegas, or an odd feeling of reckless abandon. I'm not sure, but words just burst out of me. He was peacefully minding his own business, soaking up the sun, when I approached him. My white bikini reflected back at me in his glasses as I stopped and looked straight at him.

"Well, look at you sitting there with your great arms and abs, thinking you're hot shit," I said.

The moment the words left my lips, I couldn't believe what I had just said. I'll never know exactly what came over me that day. I had never spoken to anyone like that, especially someone I didn't know. I can be direct and bold at times, but that was way out of character even for me. My friendliness had turned a bit overzealous, and I quickly realized I was way out of line.

Before I could apologize, he calmly smirked at me; I was certain a well-deserved tongue-lashing was coming my way. Whatever he was going to say, I knew I had it coming. My direct words had caught his attention, and he took off his sunglasses to reveal piercing blue eyes. I slowly removed my sunglasses to uncover my dark brown eyes and blushed with embarrassment.

"What did you just say?"

His question seemed to hang in the air momentarily as I gathered my thoughts. I couldn't possibly repeat the words I'd said only seconds before, let alone admit I'd said them. I was far too mortified by the sudden brazenness I had found in Vegas. Lowering my head slightly, I was speechless as I waited for a well-deserved verbal beating.

"If you have enough nerve to say that to me, then I need to get to know the girl that thinks I'm hot shit," he said coolly.

I watched in surprise as he slowly put his beer down on the hot concrete and slid into the pool. He confidently walked over to me and towered over my petite frame. Embarrassed, an apology couldn't come out fast enough.

"I am so sorry. I have no idea why I said that. It is so out of character for me. I mean, you are hot, but my apologies for being so forward and disrespectful. I don't know what came over me." Intrigued by my boldness, he began the introductions.

Four hours and a bucket of beers later, we had spent the entire afternoon giggling at my audacious choice of words as we got to know each other. His name was Jeff, the same as my brother Jeff, who had died of cancer when I was in my twenties. There were many differences at first glance, but the attraction was immediate; it was palpable. Once we exchanged the basics, we discovered that we both loved country music and sports, had a deep-rooted faith that anchored us, and had strong family ties. We were born the same year, just six weeks apart. He was the youngest of four children, just like me, with his siblings comprising three daughters and one son, just like mine. He had lost his father recently to an illness, and I had lost my brother Jeff after a brutal twelve-year battle with cancer in 1995.

Through hours of conversation, it became far more than Vegas pool chatter and flirting. We both started to feel a strange pull toward each other. As Jeff stood next to me in the pool, suddenly, our pinkie fingers found each other under the water. The feeling of his touch was so simple, but it had an enormous impact. My heart missed a beat, and I felt as though I had known him for years. It was warm and welcoming; I never wanted to let go, and apparently, neither did he.

Walking me to the bathroom later that day, he held my pinkie to the door, only letting go for a minute when I walked in. He immediately grabbed it again when I came out, and I knew he must have felt the same magnetic pull. That afternoon, hours in the pool were filled with laughter, sharing stories of how we were both the youngest in a family with four children, our travels all over the world, the pain we'd endured, and our passions and dreams. The sun was beginning to set, but we couldn't absorb enough of each other, both of us wanting to share and learn more. There were no awkward pauses but rather long pauses of simply gazing at each other, breathing in everything from the smell of sunscreen to the fresh vibrancy of a new relationship.

That's where my girlfriends found me, at the other end of the pool, in deep conversation with a strange man when it was time to get ready for our last night in Vegas. I didn't want to leave; everything in me wanted to stay with him and blow off my friends. It seemed impossible that in Vegas, one of the busiest and loneliest cities, I had found Jeff and made such an authentic, soulful connection. Not wanting to delay our group any longer, as I could see the rightful irritation, Jeff asked for my number. I hadn't been in the dating scene since my early twenties, over twenty years ago, so it seemed like the smart, safe thing to do was to ask for his number instead of giving him mine. Still holding his pinkie, I looked up from the pool, pleadingly at the birthday girl. Slightly annoyed, she pushed her feelings aside for me and said, "I'll put his number in my phone."

For some reason, Jeff didn't think Heather was actually typing when he gave her his number. He asked Heather for her phone so he could type his number in himself and ensure it was typed correctly. She obliged.

Throughout that last night with the girls, I could feel excitement slowly building inside me. It started at dinner, my mind drifting between the conversation with my girlfriends and those piercing blue eyes in the pool. Thoughts of Jeff and our conversation continued to pop into my mind as my excitement increased after dinner and through the end of the Britney Spears concert. Not being a Britney fan, I tried my best to be in the moment and enjoy myself at the concert for the sake of my friends. I felt restless and excited as it finally concluded. For me, the concert couldn't finish quickly enough.

As the evening finally drew to a close, I could hardly wait, knowing I would soon text Jeff to meet for a drink. I wanted to spend more time getting to know him before leaving in the morning, Jeff for Canada, and me for Los Angeles. On the walk back to our hotel, I felt like I was floating above the sidewalk. Butterflies filled my stomach, and thoughts of my evening ahead with Jeff raced through my mind. I asked Heather for his number so I could message him. She looked at me resolutely.

"I deleted it. You told me you didn't want to make a Vegas mistake."

Her response blindsided me, and a strong wave of painful disappointment washed over me. I was irritated that she deleted his number, but more than that, I was crushed to think that I would never see him again. My heart filled with a deep aching that didn't make sense; I'd only met the man that afternoon. But the pull was so intense that I couldn't hide my disappointment.

There was silence for a moment as her words hung in the air, heavy and impossible to process. Slowly, I let the disappointment sink in and permeate every inch of me. She had deleted Jeff's number. I couldn't believe it. I wasn't looking for anything I would regret; I sincerely just wanted to spend more time getting to know him. Rather than get mad at the birthday girl, I tried convincing myself that she was right. I decided to move on and asked her to watch for Jeff. Maybe I'd get lucky twice in Vegas. I forced myself to let it go as we continued to enjoy our last night in Vegas with the girls, having a great time. But all night, my thoughts drifted back to Jeff; I couldn't get him off my mind.

Sharing the suite with the birthday girl, we woke up and lay in bed the following day. We giggled and reminisced, exchanging stories of the wonderful long weekend. We began to get ready for the airport, and I looked over at Heather, still slightly disappointed. I explained that I still couldn't believe she had deleted Jeff's number. Frustrated, like a lovesick teenager, I told my friend that there had been something magical between us. I wasn't upset, just disappointed at the lost opportunity. Heather looked at me with a devilish smile and asked if I really liked him.

"Yes!" I exclaimed.

There was something there that I couldn't explain. I felt so alive. Not wanting to end her wonderful birthday weekend on a sour note, I thanked her for being a great friend and told her not to worry. Following a lengthy pause, she turned to me.

"Well … if you really like this guy, here's his number."

I exclaimed, "What, you kept it?!"

I was thrilled. I thought his number was lost forever, and we would never see each other again. Thanking her, I couldn't text his number fast enough. Immediately, the blue bubble popped back up, wondering what happened to me last night, as he told me he was waiting with his phone charging at a Starbucks to be on Wi-Fi in case I texted. I quickly explained what happened, and then we shared how excited we were to connect again. Realizing the time, I had to pack, shower, and get to the airport. Jeff asked if he could meet me downstairs and carry my bag to the taxi.

"Yes, of course," I said, thinking he was a gentleman.

I couldn't wait to see him. I stood with my bag in the lobby, waiting for him to meet me. When I saw him eagerly walking toward me, the powerful connection I'd remembered all night hit once more. It was instantly familiar and magical as his eyes met mine, and my heart raced. I felt like I had finally found my home, and it was with him. His lips parted to reveal a huge, gleaming white smile. His long gait sped up, and we half ran through the lobby toward each other, meeting in a deep embrace. Warm relief spread through me. I thought I'd never see him again, but now everything had changed, and my world felt full of promise. Holding hands and waiting together for the taxi, my stomach tightened, and a wave of nausea swept over me. I didn't want to let go. I didn't want to leave him, but I had to say goodbye and get on my plane back to Los Angeles. Jeff's flight to Canada was set to leave later that evening. As our eyes locked, the worry began to set in, and the longing for each other started. I could feel the youthful glow inside me begin to ignite and flicker fast, feeling tingly and anxious. I could feel the electricity stirring inside me; what had been asleep for years had awakened. He was a stranger less than twenty-four hours earlier. But after a few short hours together, his touch felt like something I couldn't live without.

Next to the taxi, we hugged tightly, our hearts in agony, knowing the vast distance that would soon lie between us. An insurmountable loneliness seemed to settle in as we realized how far apart we would be in just a few hours. Trying to be strong, we let go of each other and said goodbye as I got in the cab and prepared to leave. Just as the car pulled away from the curb, my phone lit up with a text. It was Jeff. Somehow, I knew everything would be okay.

From the first day, we never played games. If we felt it, we said it and did it. There was no holding back, regardless of the other person's reaction. That day in the cab, he texted and asked me to catch a later flight to spend a few more hours together. None were available, so we flew separately to different parts of North America that night. Little did we know then that our relationship would be an endless battle with time. The weekend I met Jeff, we brought back something unusual from Vegas: a remarkable love story. Our relationship would be filled with risks, going "all in" and never surrendering to our fears, so it's fitting that Las Vegas was where everything began.

Vegas is known for "What happens in Vegas stays in Vegas," but Jeff and I always joked that for us, "What happened in Vegas came home with us, and lasted a beautiful lifetime." What began as two strangers from separate countries living very different lives became something beautiful that neither could have expected.

We often joked about what a mismatch we were on paper. We lived in two different countries; he was Catholic, and I'm Jewish; he was Scottish-Irish, and I'm Scottish-Mexican; he was a respiratory therapist, and I'm an attorney; he was from a small hamlet outside of Edmonton, Alberta, with a population of 80, and I'm from Los Angeles. The entire population of Canada is the same as the state of California. We lived 2,000 miles apart across borders; we needed passports and major planning to see each other. We spoke for a handful of hours and said goodbye as I got into a taxi; that's all it took for us to start a whirlwind international romance.

But that's the thing about paper: it's an inanimate object. Paper isn't alive; it can't feel what the soul feels, and it doesn't speak for the heart. Paper does not feel anything, it can only state facts. For me and Jeff, what was on paper was far less important than what our hearts felt; that's what we let guide our destiny.

From the moment we first met, there were no traditional date nights like dinner and a movie. Logistically, we didn't have the time that most new couples do to spend a few hours leisurely getting to know each other throughout the week. Most couples go out for a few hours a week in the beginning. We, on the other hand, spent twenty-four hours a day together, four to seven days at a time. We often joked that in dog years, we'd been together for over fifty years. One day was like eight weeks of dating, which allowed our love to grow exponentially every week and month that passed. There were moments I questioned whether my feelings could be real; it all seemed too perfect. I cautiously vetted him, spending time investigating and verifying that he was legitimate. Over time, I began to let down my guard and opened my heart to the realization that the love I had always dreamed of truly existed.

Between planned visits to each other's countries, we spent countless hours talking and FaceTiming, discovering every detail. We familiarized ourselves with everything from our childhoods to the tiny, ordinary details of each other's daily lives. We unraveled the layers of our lives and shared intimate details. In the beginning, we were often overwhelmed with how a relationship between us could realistically work and were apprehensive if we wanted to put effort into something that may not work out.

One day, I told him, "Listen, I know it's not going to be easy what we're doing; it's not conventional, but how I see it is, 'We miss 100 percent of the shots we never take.'"

Stunned, Jeff asked, "Did you just quote the great one back to me?" Referring to Wayne Gretzky, arguably the best hockey player of all time.

I explained to Jeff that it's a quote I live by whenever I feel fear and trepidation creeping in. He not only realized I, too, was a Gretzky hockey fan, but we also lived by a similar motto. In that instant, we both decided we were all in.

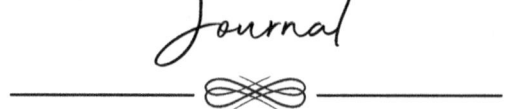

Sometimes the greatest risks are not taken in business, or on a card table, but with your own heart. When you think back on your own life, when have you taken a chance that defied logic but felt right in your soul? Write about a time you followed that inner nudge, even when the outcome was unknown.

Chapter 3

SURF AND SAND

Despite living thousands of miles apart, Jeff and I made every effort to see each other often. His first visit to see me in California solidified our relationship. Driving to pick him up from the airport, a mix of nerves and excitement swirled inside me. My hands trembled slightly, my heart pounded in my chest, and my mind raced with a thousand thoughts—what if this moment wasn't as perfect as I had imagined? The anticipation of seeing him in person for the first time had my stomach in knots. The moment our arms wrapped around each other and our lips met for the first time, all my nerves melted away. I knew I was home.

We completely absorbed every moment we shared; each visit was a lifeline tethering us more tightly until the next visit. There was a strong, never-ending tug at our hearts, but we had no plan. The seemingly irrational behavior of two very structured and logical people was anything but normal for us. It made sense that our loved ones initially found our unusual behavior challenging to understand. We moved forward, not listening to the naysayers, refusing to let anything get in the way of the love we knew we shared. We were confident we could make it work; we had to take it one day and one conversation at a time.

We both had careers and full lives. Nothing about our new situation was familiar, and it would not be easy. But we knew we would do whatever was necessary to find time together, often flying three hours one way only to spend twenty-four hours together before heading back to the airport. The pattern would be repeated dozens of times yearly for over three and a half years. Each visit allowed our hearts to find each other and reconnect until the next visit. We racked up airline miles as logic took a back seat, and we let our hearts guide us. I would not advise anyone to take such a path, but for some reason, that illogical way of living for the first half of our relationship made perfect sense to us. Over time, it was undeniable that everyone could see what we knew and felt.

On one of Jeff's visits to California, I surprised him with a birthday stay at The Surf and Sand Hotel in Laguna Beach. It was our first time at the exceptional property. Living in Southern California, I had heard how spectacular the resort was, so I was excited to share the unique experience with Jeff.

The hotel is located directly on the beach, with spectacular ocean sunset views. The pool is set just above the sand, with glass walls overlooking the ocean. The entire property, from the moment you enter the lobby to the beautifully decorated rooms, is filled with relaxation and romance at every turn, making one feel incredibly spoiled.

When I picked Jeff up at LAX, I couldn't stop the car fast enough. I wanted nothing more than to hold and kiss him. The agonizing build-up of only speaking for weeks over FaceTime and phone calls made seeing each other again feel like it was the first time. As I pulled up to the curbside at LAX to pick him up that day, excitement bubbled inside me. It had been only a few weeks since we tearfully said goodbye at the airport in Canada, but since that time, the roller-coaster of highs and lows had brought me to a point of desperation to see him once more. The exhilaration of knowing we would spend the next several days together, connecting in such a romantic setting, felt magical.

I quickly put the car in park, anticipation bursting. I couldn't wait to hold the man I had fallen deeply in love with. Jeff stood on the curb in flip-flops, wearing a soft, mint-green t-shirt, ready for some sunshine. He excitedly waved, a smile beaming across his face.

Before I could open my door, he was already running for me, his light brown hair framing bright blue eyes that pierced into me. He looked so handsome with a chiseled jawline that fell below his full lips as he swiftly moved his long, lean, muscular frame. He left his luggage at the curb, threw open my door, and pulled me out of the car. Lifting me into his strong arms, we held onto each other like it was our last time. Lost in each other, we stood embracing and kissing. Time stood still. With car horns blaring, jets taking flight, families bustling, and yelling all around us. It all fell away, and the world went silent. Somehow, all I could smell was the musk on his neck, feel the warmth in his embrace, hear the depth of his voice, and taste forever on my lips.

We sank deeply into each other as we kissed and held on, breathing life back into our lungs.

We were lost in our blissful embrace when an elderly gentleman gently tapped Jeff on the back. Certain that he wanted us to move the car with all the heavy LAX traffic we were likely holding up; we slowly pulled away from each other and gave him our attention. Glancing up, Jeff patiently and politely asked, "How can we help you, sir?" The gentleman responded with words I will never forget. "I want to thank you both for reminding me what love looks like. You don't see this kind of love every day. You made my week by watching your embracing love." Feeling the lightness of our love and knowing we had four days to share, Jeff and I looked at him with a smile and an inquisitive glance.

Looking back on that moment, it still bewilders me as I recall the purity of his heart in approaching two strangers and sharing that he saw what we felt in our hearts. The gentleman at LAX saw the love Jeff and I felt; what we had was palpable and raw. The airport wasn't the only time we experienced people commenting on the love they could see radiating from us. We once received surprise glasses of champagne sent to our table to "cheer us" while eating dinner. Another time, strangers asked to take our pictures because of the love they felt. Although not uncommon for us, it was a strange phenomenon, but the most memorable of all occurred that weekend while staying at the Surf and Sand Hotel in Laguna Beach.

We checked into our room, which was no ordinary room. The room was beautifully appointed with soft ocean blues, pillowy clouds of white everywhere, and touches of the sea in every décor. The hotel had perfectly named it the "drop a penny in the sand room." Once settled, we learned quickly what that term meant. Walking onto the balcony, we saw that we could effortlessly drop a penny into the beach surf and sand below. Standing four stories up, the sea's salt and the ocean's roar overpowered our senses before we saw it. An endless view of waves and countless dreams to explore stretched before us as we gazed out over the beach. We stood on our balcony that afternoon and looked down as the ocean waves slowly painted the sand below with layers of tiny seashells. We listened as each wave brought the sound of a beating heart and new life while we enjoyed a glass of wine, breathing in the anticipation of the next four days together.

Jeff was never in a hurry; he loved to enjoy each moment and experience. He intentionally made time for the most important things in life, especially when making memories. Being raised in the Los Angeles area, slow did not come naturally for me, but I learned to embrace this beautiful new lens through which to view and experience life. It was one of his qualities I loved. He was a master at taking his time with every conversation and every experience. In a world where we plan and hurry, Jeff and I controlled our environment by slowing everything down and capturing every scent and feeling we could absorb. It was in those moments when unexpected encounters pleasantly captured our hearts.

It was early in the day, and after sitting on our balcony and enjoying the ocean views, we made a dinner reservation to watch the sunset at the restaurant and then made our way down to the pool. We spent the following few hours sharing our life's dreams as we frolicked in the pool and took walks on the beach. We fell deeper in love with each other. Touching pinkies, we reminisced on our first meeting in the Vegas pool and dreamt of the day we would live together. Locked in our bubble, we didn't notice anyone around us. We weren't impolite; we were in our own world and didn't want to lose a single minute. It was as if our hearts somehow knew what we didn't, that time was limited, and we had to make each moment meaningful.

We soon realized the hours had passed too quickly and had to move our dinner reservation to make it on time. The sun was setting, so we rearranged our evening to watch the sunset from our balcony and then get ready for dinner. Moving reservations and showing up late had become a common theme in our relationship as we often got caught up in each other's deep blues and dark browns. In our relationship, we welcomed the unexpected, allowing unforgettable moments to trickle in and reshape our plans. It wasn't about the schedule but the memories we were creating along the way.

With all our belongings, we left the pool and waited for the elevator. The door opened, and a precious little girl exited with her mom. Dressed in a floral sundress and summer sandals, she had big brown eyes framed by long brown hair with curls and bows. Kneeling to her eye level, Jeff and I told her how beautiful she looked in her dress for dinner that night and wished her and her mom a lovely evening. We had missed the elevator as we got caught up in visiting with the little girl. We could hear her talking to her mom while waiting for the next elevator, still in our swimsuits and pool hats. She softly said in a sweet, pure voice, "Mommy, that's the prince and princess from the pool." Jeff and I looked back at the mom inquisitively, and she told us something that perfectly explained how our hearts felt. The mom said, "My daughter was watching you all day at the pool and told me you were both a prince and a princess. In her purest of eyes, she saw a fairytale of what she thought a happily ever after looked like." We melted. How could this young heart see what we felt? We just looked at the mom and little girl, speechless for a moment. Finally, I said, "Thank you." Jeff and I bent down again and said, "Sweetie, that is so incredibly special, and we want to thank you so much for sharing your heart with us." Elevators continued to pass us by as we became lost in conversation with the child and her mother.

I now realize that it wasn't a coincidence that an elderly gentleman at LAX and a child in Laguna Beach each captured our love through their eyes and shared it with us. Our love was palpable. Looking back, I am so grateful that they openly expressed what they witnessed; it gave me a lifetime of loving memories to hold onto that I didn't know I needed to lock away for what our future held. Because of our circumstances, living so far apart and not knowing when or if we would ever live together, Jeff and I chose to live each day intentionally. We found purpose in the time we shared, learning to compartmentalize the sadness that loomed, knowing we would inevitably have to drive back to the airport and say goodbye.

Soaking in that sweet child's words, we returned to our room and canceled our dinner reservation. Instead, we ordered room service and sat on the balcony all evening, watching the moonlight turn into the sunrise.

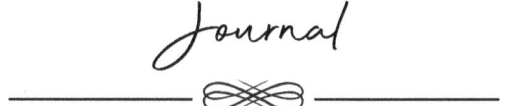

Some moments in life are so pure, so saturated with love, that even strangers can feel them. Those are the moments worth slowing down for, savoring, and tucking away in your soul. Think about a time when you were fully present with someone you love, so much so that the outside world seemed to pause. What details, sights, sounds, and feelings do you remember most vividly from that moment?

Chapter 4
TOGETHER

I knew I had met my forever life partner, and the last piece of our puzzle was how and when to blend our lives. We had been dating for three years, what felt like an eternity, when Jeff offered to move to California. Having dedicated twenty-eight years in the ICU at The Alec in Edmonton, Jeff decided it was time to retire his stethoscope. He considered our situations and what made the most sense under the circumstances. My son, Jake, who was in high school, still lived at home, but my daughter Maddie and Jeff's two children had all moved out. Having discussed it thoroughly, we concluded that our options were to wait until Jake graduated from high school in two years or for Jeff to move to California sooner. Tension had been building for a while as we became increasingly frustrated, not knowing when or if we would ever live together in the same country. Feeling the emotional strain of a long-term, long-distance relationship, Jeff decided to move to California. Additionally, he was excited to leave behind the bitterly cold Canadian winters for California's year-round sunshine.

The U-Haul was securely fastened to the back of the GMC truck; there wasn't an inch of room remaining inside. Like most things, Jeff took great care in ensuring that all his precious belongings, from photos to hockey memorabilia, his beloved barbecue, and his Canadian Lamb's rum, which he mixed with Canada Dry for his favorite cocktail, were tightly cinched down. Everything was packed up perfectly for the start of our new life. We were beyond excited—three years had passed, and we could finally wake up together every day for the rest of our lives. We were brimming with excitement and anticipation for all the years of memories that lay ahead of us.

We could never have known the obstacles we overcame the past few years paled in comparison to the road that lay before us.

The life-altering decision to move involved so many emotions. Since grade school, Jeff's life had been in Edmonton and the surrounding areas. He was leaving his home, carrying decades of memories locked away in his heart, so that we could live life together in California. When Jeff offered to move to the States, it was thoughtful and romantic, but also very complex. Other hearts and loved ones were involved, which had to be considered.

Everyone was happy for us; they knew how challenging it was for Jeff and me to live apart, and we appreciated everyone's loving support. There were many tearful goodbyes and long embraces next to the truck as Jeff's friends and family gathered to send us off. Making a permanent move to another country was a courageous act that involved sacrifices.

During the four-day drive south, we reminisced about the last few years and how we loved spending time with each other's families in our respective countries as we became integral parts of each other's lives. Although we cherished the memories of intertwining our lives, we were emotionally worn out from years of coordinating work and kids' schedules every few weeks so that one of us could fly to meet the other.

The endless cycle of long goodbyes at airports every few weeks over the past three years was filled with heavy sadness and tears that tore at our hearts. Our visits had been lined with so many conflicting feelings. Leading up to each of our trips, we were like restless, giddy, young school kids in love, the enthusiasm written on our faces. Jeff said that his coworkers at The Alec always knew when we would see each other or when we had just said a tearful goodbye at the airport; he was either elated and joyful or tense and agitated. We couldn't hide the heavy emotions we were living with. Each trip brought us closer, deepening our understanding of each other. Everything felt natural—except the miles that separated us. Only one thing was missing: living daily life side by side.

The extensive planning was also very taxing on us; we just wanted to be together, to fall asleep in each other's arms and wake up to each other. Our patience was wearing thin, and Jeff's temper flared up more frequently as he became increasingly irritated at the unknown timeframe that remained for us living apart. During the last twenty-four hours of each visit, as we began packing bags to return to our own country, a heavy melancholy would set in, and we both fought to enjoy those last hours together.

On one visit in particular, Jeff planned for us to go quad-riding in Radium, a small, quiet town in eastern British Columbia. We loaded the truck and made the six-hour drive down from Edmonton, meandering our way past Canmore and Banff through the Canadian Rockies, enjoying a front-row view of stunning natural beauty. It was the beginning of fall, just before winter would cover the land with a cool, white blanket. Spectacular views surrounded us the entire drive: countless acres of open ranges with endless fields of thick grassland swaying in the wind between the dotted, floral accents of pink, orange, and purple wildflowers. Meanwhile, the stately elk and moose grazed in their natural habitat as we drove past.

Viewing the magnificent Three Sisters Mountain peaks, we smiled at the irony of three sisters in each of our families. The Three Sisters in Canmore are the town's most recognizable majestic peaks. With their high elevation and sharp, jagged edges, each one is slightly higher than the next. The rugged terrain was covered with a dusting of snow, revealing the immense power of nature, all easily viewed from the highway. Driving past glass-like, crystal clear lakes, the fragrance of spruce and fir trees filled my senses with each breath, and I was captivated by the endless sea of fragrant trees clinging to the mountain ranges. Watching the elk, deer, and moose roam freely was genuinely spectacular to this California girl.

As we made our way closer to Radium, the Sinclair Mountain Pass rose ahead of us on Highway 93. As it loomed closer, the breathtaking views led us through the rocky walls of the steep, towering orange and grey canyons that the highway sharply cut through. The cliff's edges towered over the truck on both sides of the road while water spilled into the deep canyon below. Jeff was rightfully proud to share the splendor of his homeland—it was breathtaking. Listening to our favorite country tunes and soaking in the beauty while we fell more in love at every turn of the road, I loved everything about that man and his beautiful country.

It was his birthday, and we planned a romantic weekend in a condo where we barbecued, sipped wine on the patio, and took long walks watching the sunset. On one of my prior visits, Jeff introduced me to his favorite treat, a Canadian dessert called Nanaimo bars. The delicious, sweet treat originated in Nanaimo, British Columbia. It consisted of a coconut and nut crumb base, custard filling, and a layer of chocolate ganache. Jeff was not a big dessert or sweets lover, but he loved Nanaimo bars primarily because of the coconut base, one of his favorite flavors.

I packed all the ingredients for the mouthwatering bars in my suitcase and surprised him by making them for his birthday. I remember that night in the kitchen, how he watched admiringly and grabbed me periodically for a slow dance, saying with the most genuine care in his voice, "No one has ever made me homemade Nanaimo bars, Honeybee; I can't believe you remembered." I didn't realize the impact the small gesture had on him. He repeatedly mentioned how impressed he was that I made the bars for him; you would have thought I won the national baking contest. But to Jeff, it was always the simplest things in life that he truly appreciated and valued. Never short on compliments, he let me know the gratitude in his heart. Yes, they were delicious, but he was more taken aback that I had remembered him mentioning the bars months prior and that I packed the ingredients up to Canada. These small moments of appreciation and his sincere expressions of love were so endearing to me. The seemingly ordinary moments connected us deeply, as we were never afraid to express our feelings. Nothing was taken for granted or lost on us.

It was a wonderful birthday dinner celebration, making Jeff his favorite Mexican dishes. We still had two more days together to explore the outdoors of British Columbia and the quaint surrounding town, continually filling our souls to withstand the miles between us. We uncovered more layers of our relationship while discovering the Radium hot springs and the natural beauty of the first signs of fall. On one of the days in Radium, we went quadding through the beautiful trails lined with the yellow larch trees, taking turns driving while the other hung on with our arms tightly wrapped around, racing through streams and soaking in the fresh mountain air. Jeff packed a picnic with an assortment of cheese and wine for an adventurous day in the breathtaking wilderness. We set up a table on the back of the quad, playfully sipped, and snacked, appreciating the scenic backdrop and how fortunate we were to have found each other. With our picnic next to us, we relished another unforgettable weekend.

Making our way back to the condo, the dark clouds rolling across the Canadian skies mimicked our gloomy moods. Our emotions changed almost instantly as we left our picnic behind, knowing the next day we'd make the drive back to the Calgary airport. From there, Jeff would have another three-hour drive back to Edmonton while I flew the three hours back to Los Angeles.

The following day, we headed to the airport, feeling sullen. On the drive, I could see Jeff was becoming increasingly miserable. The mood in the truck was the opposite of when he had picked me up at the airport just days earlier. The drive was entirely void of laughter and playfulness. Holding hands, I looked his way just as his brows began to furrow and tears slowly etched soft lines down his cheeks. He stopped in Canmore for fuel, an hour and a half from the Calgary airport, and I could feel the knots in my stomach tighten as we inched closer to another dreaded goodbye. Outside, Jeff filled the tank. I could see his head down as he wiped away tears. The familiar, miserable feeling that led to melancholy had come back. He returned to the truck and sorrowfully said, "Honeybee, how will we keep doing this? Can we sustain this? How long do you think we'll have to continue living apart?" Neither of us had an answer; all we knew was that we were both fully committed to making our relationship work.

Jeff slowly pulled out of the service station, and once again, we began making the heart-wrenching trek to the airport. A deafening silence had settled into the truck's cab as we both tried to deal with the reality of another blissful weekend ending too soon. That is when the truck began to sputter and make a knocking sound. Jeff pulled to the side of the road, his pain and heartache quickly turning into a mouth full of curse words. "Shit!" he yelled out. "Never in my life have I ever made that mistake. I'm so fuckin' pissed at myself right now!" He exclaimed, "I put in regular fuel instead of diesel; I wasn't paying attention."

He knew if he continued to drive with the wrong fuel, he would ruin the engine. We needed a tow to a mechanic who could drain and flush the truck's fuel tank. We called AMA (Canada's AAA) and waited patiently on the side of the highway for a tow to Calgary. My flight departed as we got a ride in the tow truck. This would not be the only flight missed; it was just one more time Jeff and I struggled to make our worlds fit.

We dropped the truck off for repair and took an Uber to the airport, hoping to find another flight, but there were none. Recognizing we were stuck, we looked at each other, and the anger of the truck fiasco, along with the sorrow in our hearts, melted away. Smiles washed over our faces as we delighted in the sudden realization that we had received a gift; Jeff's error extended our time together. We decided to make the most of the fifteen hours together before my flight the following day. We called every hotel near the airport and learned they were all full. Exasperated but determined, we walked to the Delta Hotel attached to the airport terminal. Explaining our predicament to a woman at the front desk, we begged her to look for any room. The friendly Canadian clerk stepped aside to speak with her manager. Upon returning, she said in a peculiar tone, "Well, I do have one room, but we don't typically rent it out." We thought that was odd, but as long as it was clean and safe, we didn't care. The clerk handed us the key with detailed instructions on how to find and access the room, and we proceeded to the hotel's lowest level.

Walking past several conference rooms, we came to a small door without a room number, located where the clerk had told us it would be. The room we stepped into was more like a basement. Our eyes quickly scanned the windowless space with a Murphy bed folded up against the far wall and a shiny pole in the middle of the room, which was firmly affixed from the floor to the ceiling. Simultaneously Jeff and I burst out laughing hysterically. Our minds had reached the same conclusion that the room was clearly for stripper parties.

Grateful to have another night together, regardless of the strange room we had found ourselves in, we grabbed a bottle of wine from the bar upstairs and lay in the very uncomfortable Murphy bed in a room with no views, giggling at the irony of that day. The laughter was a much-needed stress relief from the day we'd had. The extra time somehow made the next day one of our easiest goodbyes.

Although his roots were deeply embedded in Canadian soil, Jeff would quickly become accustomed to the California lifestyle, which suited him. I knew I was the luckiest girl in the world, in part because he was devilishly handsome with a beautifully toned physique, but I loved his confidence in knowing what made him happy. Jeff was never afraid to live in the moment. Life beside him felt right.

As we drove the U-Haul hooked up to the truck those two thousand miles, we became acutely aware that only three highways had divided us over the last three years. Although that suddenly seemed minor to us, the distance and time apart had grown increasingly unbearable with each passing year. We drove through each state, winding our way toward our new future and enjoying the beauty surrounding us.

Driving into Yellowstone National Park, we marveled at the buffalo and other wildlife roaming outside our windows. We enjoyed endless hours on the road, passionately sharing our hopes and dreams for all that lay ahead.

The excitement overflowed as we turned the corner onto our street and pulled into our driveway, seeing our forever home together. Although we had spent so much time together in that home over the past few years, as we walked over the welcome mat and opened the door, it finally felt like we were truly home. Looking around, we relished all the details Jeff helped me choose to design the home I had purchased when we first met. We could see it all come together, from the kitchen and lighting fixtures to the landscape and pool. It was now our time to build a future together. We spent the next week unloading Jeff's belongings and weaving them into our home, imagining all the years ahead with endless opportunities to create a lifetime of memories together.

When Jeff moved to California, we were both forty-eight years old and had our entire lives ahead of us. We spent the next year enjoying being together daily and growing even closer. Jeff had a deep love for California and its golden coastlines, but he needed something to keep him busy and replace the career he had left. He spent most days researching business opportunities where we could work together. He also looked at some viable work options, including working as a traveling respiratory therapist. I had taken fifteen years off to raise children and recently returned to the same law firm where I had previously practiced. As in-house defense counsel for Liberty Mutual Insurance Company, I became painfully aware that although I was successful, I wasn't happy practicing law anymore. Something had shifted inside me, and although I once loved practicing law, I now felt disconnected from it.

As a lawyer and a respiratory therapist, our careers had been filled with intensity and unhappiness. People didn't come to our places of business if life was good. Jeff had cared for patients in the ICU, and witnessing life and death daily took a sizeable mental toll on him over the years. In my career, I represented clients when they were being sued, and I was under extreme pressure. By the end of that first year, we both realized that neither of our careers suited what we desired in life: to find joy in each day.

We wanted to enjoy the second half of our lives together in a more pleasant and relaxed atmosphere. With three kids in college plus regular life expenses, retiring was not an option. We knew we'd need to find a new career that would suit us both and where we could work together, so looking for a business to purchase seemed like a great idea.

From the first day we met in Vegas, we took countless risks to be together. For us, taking calculated risks was a better approach to life than sitting back and letting life happen to us. Neither of us wanted to look back on life and wonder, "What if we had only..." Instead, we both held immense value in living a life of no regrets. We had responsibilities, but taking calculated risks was built into our cores. We were both risk- takers with boundaries; for us, it was a perfect life partnership.

Shortly before Jeff moved to California, we planned a family trip with our four children to visit my nieces in Chicago. While there, Jeff surprised me with a beautiful proposal. Shortly after our engagement, I received an email from a production studio looking to cast aspiring business owners who wanted to take a leap of faith in a reality show titled *Buy Your Own Business (BYOB)*. *Seriously?* I thought. What are the chances that, as we were looking to buy a business, this TV show was looking for couples to interview and cast for precisely that? I had an invention over a dozen years ago and was on an inventor TV show with my product. That show must have put my contact information into a database because I had received many casting emails over the years. The email from *BYOB* was the first one I answered. Being on a TV show was the farthest thing from our minds, but if it was an avenue for the means to our end, why not apply? At first glance, we both had no interest. But with us, life was always an adventure, so we thought, *What the hell?* I emailed the casting director, shared our story, and provided the requested pictures and why we wanted to buy a business. Two days later, I received an email asking Jeff and I to send in a video submission by answering some prompts so they could see and hear us on film. Over the next five months, we filled out multiple forms, were given background checks, and participated in Skype interviews.

Following months of interviews, the producer called to tell us we were chosen to film the show. We were shocked and excited, realizing what a long shot it was to get cast. We couldn't believe we had been selected. Once again, we threw caution to the wind and accepted the opportunity to find a business on a TV show. Over a few months, the production team followed and filmed us while the show's host presented us with three business options within our parameters. They filmed us visiting each business, meeting the owners, and asking questions. We chose to buy one of the businesses, which was near the beach and closer to where we wanted to move one day.

There were bills to be paid, so while Jeff and I filmed the show looking for a business to purchase, I continued my career as an attorney. During that time, I began preparing for an extensive trial. When the trial started in a downtown Los Angeles courtroom, Jeff came daily to support me, cheering me on from the gallery just as he had at the half-marathon I ran on my first trip to Canada. He sat intently from jury selection until the jurors returned with a verdict. I loved feeling his unassuming strength from the gallery. At the end of the two-week trial, we met with friends at a bar in downtown Los Angeles to celebrate my 12-0 defense verdict. The following week, I gave my two-week notice.

Suddenly, our new joint career began. We were now the proud owners of a hair salon in Laguna Hills, a forty-five-minute drive from our home in Chino Hills. Neither of us was a hair stylist, but growing up watching our parents run their businesses, we instinctively knew we could run this business successfully. It provided us with what we wanted: a steady income, a new career filled with clients who left happier than when they walked in, and the opportunity for me and Jeff to work together every day.

Many of our friends and family thought we were crazy for buying a hair salon, but they knew we'd been unconventional together since the day we met, so it made perfect sense. With the business in full swing, we were thrilled to finally make up for all the years of lost time; now, we could spend every day together.

We walked into ownership in January 2018 with our hearts full. Everything was complete; we spent the past three and a half years setting the stage for a beautiful life we knew was ahead. We would work together daily at our new business, take drives down to the beach from work, make plans to one day move to the beach, enjoy all the kids as they grew into adulthood, and continue to fall deeper in love. The years of patiently waiting and planning had led up to that moment when everything finally came to fruition. Little did we know how taking risks and going "all in" would be useful for the life ahead we couldn't see. What was lying beneath the surface would soon drastically change our lives.

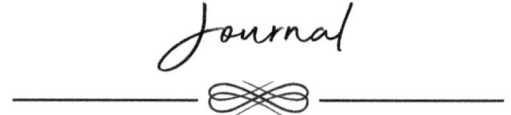

Sometimes love asks us to take leaps that look risky on paper but feel certain in the heart. Those leaps can change everything. Think of a time when you or someone you love made a major life decision in the name of love, partnership, or shared dreams. What fears did you have to push through, and what gave you the courage to take that step?

Chapter 5

NEW BEGINNINGS

We started the new year with great hope and a euphoric optimism engulfing our souls. Toasting over champagne and cuddling in a low-lit corner booth, our world felt complete as January 1, 2018, arrived. Our new, carefully crafted lives were blossoming just as we had planned and hoped for. The pieces of our complicated puzzle fit perfectly together. Each tongue and groove we patiently arranged created a beautiful foundation to build our future. It had been six months since Jeff moved from Canada to California, and life felt ordinary yet extraordinary.

Everything we took risks on, from Vegas to dating three years long distance, leaving our careers to buy a business, was all paying off. Looking at any piece individually, the odds were stacked against us. We were all in from that first pinkie touch in the pool. If either of us had faltered at any time over the years, if we had given up hope or the fight to make it work, we would be just another Vegas story. It was 2018, three and a half years since we'd first met, and our dream had become a reality. We felt invincible.

We drove to and from work each day, holding hands and listening to our favorite country tunes. We enjoyed getting to know all our stylists and clients. It was exactly what we'd envisioned. It was work, of course, but it was a place everyone left happier than when they'd come in. We were in awe of how all our efforts and determination guided everything to fall into place perfectly.

On Valentine's Day that year, Jeff developed a minor sinus infection. Taking over-the-counter medications for a few weeks, his infection was not improving, and he was feeling some discomfort. We went to our general practitioner, and she gave Jeff a prescription for his symptoms, hoping that more potent medications would alleviate the pressure he was feeling. He had been miserable coming into work as his pain and discomfort continued to worsen, but he did his best to put on a happy face; he never wanted to make a fuss.

The sinus infection became terribly annoying and uncomfortable, and continued for a month. He began to stay home from work a few days each week to rest, but there was no marked improvement. In an attempt to ease his symptoms, our doctor prescribed antibiotics. By late March, I was going to work alone most days, giving Jeff time to rest, hoping I would come home each day to see some improvement. I missed having him at work and on the long drives, but I knew he was miserable and needed some time to heal.

The antibiotics brought no marked change, so our doctor put Jeff on steroids to see if that could improve his symptoms. By that time, Jeff had begun to feel some facial pain and pressure and was having frequent headaches. He also started to have slightly blurry vision in his right eye, which was attributed to the steroids. There was no improvement. We allowed our minds to consider a variety of explanations for all his stubborn symptoms. We thought Jeff's history with polyps (non-cancerous growths that lined his nasal passage) may have played a role in the persistent sinus issues. Knowing it could take some time for the steroids to address his symptoms fully, we patiently waited. We were almost two months without relief. With Jeff's medical background, and doing some research, we were sure the nasty sinus infection would eventually pass. Trying to reassure ourselves, we learned that sinus infections can often go on for extended periods. We naturally assumed Jeff's case was particularly severe.

Jeff and I loved any opportunity to spend time with either of our families. We had moved my daughter Maddie into her dorm the previous summer for her first year at college. We loved every minute of the freshman firsts, including setting up her dorm room together, putting up all her wall décor and twinkle lights, and exploring the city. In the spring, Maddie was playing college softball in Philadelphia, and we planned a trip to catch one of her last games. Even though he still wasn't feeling well, Jeff insisted on going. He didn't want to miss seeing Maddie on the field and wanted to support all her dedication and effort to play college ball. Jeff was not himself during the weekend getaway, and I could tell he was holding a lot in. Although I continually checked in to see how he was and what, if anything, I could do, he assured me it would pass.

From the time we caught our Uber ride back to the airport and took the six-hour flight home, I had a visceral feeling deep inside that something was very wrong. Call it instinct, intuition, or premonition. Despite not saying a word, as I didn't want Jeff to carry the burden of what my inner voice was telling me, I somehow found a way to quiet my apprehension. Jeff's usual, playful demeanor shifted; he was clearly in more pain than he had let on.

Within the first few days of being back in California, Jeff's blurry vision in his right eye worsened, his facial pressure and headaches became more uncomfortable, and there was still no relief. He rarely mentioned the discomfort he experienced or his inability to see out of his right eye. I didn't know how bad it was until much later. Jeff didn't want me to worry; he was the most selfless person I had ever known.

Once we had returned from Philly, he didn't come to work with me anymore. He was lethargic and visibly in pain; he just wanted to rest. He felt more tired with each passing day and lost his appetite. The aching in his head had turned into a sharp, stabbing pain, which he thought may have been caused by the flight and elevation change, possibly increasing some of the intense facial pressures he was experiencing. I went to work each day, making sure he was set up for the day at home alone. I checked on him throughout the day, hoping the latest medications would solve the persistent infection. We weren't ignoring his symptoms; it was that the rationalizations allowed our minds to choose to be optimistic and assume the best, that we would find the proper medications to offer him relief. But with each passing day, Jeff became more miserable. For over two months, the battle raged in Jeff's body, but nothing improved. Things were clearly not okay.

Long before the sun rose on April 27, 2018, Jeff woke up to penetrating pain. With the sky pitch black and the world eerily still, he leaned over to wake me. "Honeybee, I can barely see out of my right eye. Something's wrong; we need to go to the emergency room now."

Jeff would never want to go to a hospital, especially in the middle of the night, so I knew it was severe. Exhausted by lack of sleep, we stumbled around bleary-eyed as we quickly got dressed. A part of me was relieved, thinking we would finally figure out what was going on with his sinus infection.

I drove twenty-five minutes through quiet, moonlit roads to St. Jude's in Fullerton. I dropped him off to check in at the emergency room while I parked the car. By that time, we'd convinced ourselves that the nasal polyps that had been removed years earlier must have been the cause, since none of the medications were working to fix what we all thought was a terrible sinus infection.

Since our situation wasn't urgent or life-threatening, we had to wait two hours to be seen by a doctor. I was more tired than worried, knowing that Jeff worked in the ICU as a respiratory therapist for twenty-eight years. I felt he would have shown more fear if it were serious. I decided not to worry until there was something to worry about, and Jeff seemed to feel the same. He kept saying, "I'm sure it has something to do with my prior sinus infections, and this is just worse than the others. We'll figure it out."

We distracted ourselves with small talk, getting a few moments of shut-eye, leaning into each other in the chairs as we sat in the waiting room watching the sunrise as the hustle and bustle of the hospital began to filter in. Finally, we got called to the back. My mind was split between wondering what they would give Jeff so he could get rid of his sinus infection and what time we would leave so I could drive him home and make my way over to our business. I figured everything would get sorted out shortly.

They took Jeff's vitals as we explained all of his symptoms and treatments he experienced over the past couple of months. The doctor decided to order several tests, including X-rays. Once the battery of tests had been concluded, we were frustrated when nothing was revealed. Feeling discouraged and tired, we just wanted a prescription so we could go home. The doctors were equally bothered that they couldn't determine what was causing the vision issues and intense head and facial discomfort, so they decided to do a CT scan. It was now 10:00 a.m., and we had been in the hospital for over six hours. They put us in a private room to prepare Jeff for the CT scan.

The nurses prepared to wheel Jeff out for the scan. I gave him a long, soft kiss and casually said, "Everything is fine, honey; I'll see you soon." Waiting for him in the room, I started sending a couple of texts to get the work day started and began to figure out what the day would look like when the scan results came back.

Soon, he was wheeled back into the room. Both of us were tired, so we crawled into the bed to lie beside each other while waiting for the results. We lay there cuddling into each other as we took our minds to a place of happiness, mapping out the days and months ahead. Planning time with our children, family, and friends, discussing backyard swim parties and barbecues, travel, concerts, Sunday champagne, and Caesar (Canadian version of our Bloody Mary, but much better) brunches. For the past four years, these were the ways we made memories for our hearts to hold as we spent the time falling deeper in love with each other and creating a beautiful life to carry in our hearts.

Looking back, I didn't realize how intentionally we'd been living our lives since we met. We had made every moment together matter. Living so far apart, each phone call and every minute we planned to be together was vital to our relationship. Living life fully and purposefully each day became natural for us.

We knew how lucky we were to have found each other; the love and connection we shared only grew more profound, and having met in our mid-forties, we just wanted to make up for the lost time. We still had half our lives ahead of us and wanted to take full advantage of every minute we had together. In moments of privacy, Jeff would quietly look at me and say, "Honeybee, when we grow old, and it's our time, I will have to be the one to go first; I couldn't live one day without you." I would quickly reply, "We will go at the same time to protect both our hearts." Of course, those words were not meant for today. Today, we were planning to celebrate our fiftieth birthdays together later that summer. Today, our life together was just beginning.

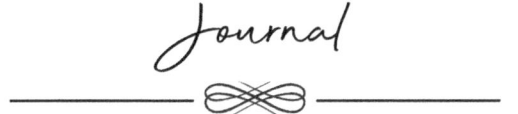

Sometimes the future changes in ways we never expect, and our perspective on what truly matters comes into sharper focus. Think about a time when life seemed perfectly on track, only to be disrupted by an unexpected challenge. How did that moment shift the way you value your time, health, or relationships?

Chapter 6

JUST BREATHE

I was lying beside Jeff, still talking, when the doctor entered the room. I looked forward to hearing the CT scan results so we could move forward with our day and enjoy the weekend. The feeling of summer was beginning, and we felt the promise of all the fun and frolicking that lay just around the corner. Sitting up in the hospital bed, we knew whatever the doctor needed to tell us would be a simple hiccup in our week and would help Jeff finally recover from his frustrating sinus issue.

"We've got the results back from your CT scan," he stated dryly.

The doctor seemed to shift uneasily for a minute before clearing his throat and moving on. I was hardly paying attention to his words, with the plans for the day and summer distracting me, when he continued.

"There's a five-centimeter tumor in your sinus region at the skull base that's intertwined and wrapped into your optic nerve."

I froze and felt Jeff tense up beside me. Suddenly, the whole world seemed to stop turning. We all know that life can change in the blink of an eye, but we never thought it would happen to us. In that instant, all our plans, hopes, and dreams evaporated. When you hear life-altering news, you are completely paralyzed. That morning, our bodies were in utter shock; we couldn't breathe or force out any words. My mind swirled frantically, and I began spiraling down a dark hole as a cold cloud of fear enveloped the room. So many questions filled every corner of my mind, but I was mute.

Was it benign or malignant? Where in the skull base, and how intertwined into the optic nerve? How big is five centimeters? (I later learned that it's the size of a lime.) Is there a treatment, and is it curable? How long do we have? How much time is left together?

I was paralyzed as I thought, *No, not again, this isn't possible.* I had already lost my brother to cancer in my twenties; he was my everything. *Not again! I can't lose Jeff too!* I screamed in my head.

Frozen, my mind was the only thing that moved; it instantly went to my brother and the terror of what that life looked like. I was only fourteen years old when my eighteen-year-old brother was diagnosed with adenoid cystic carcinoma in his right parotid gland. We were childhood and adulthood best friends; we loved doing everything together, from sports, to listening to music, debating politics, playing poker, and discussing our life's dreams and passions.

He trained with me weekly to become a top high school tennis player, ranking the number one seed in our California Interscholastic Federation division. He never allowed me to give in to my fears or doubts. There was no room for failure with my brother. There was no halfway with him. You either give everything, accept and be proud of the result, or don't bother trying. He challenged and pushed me in life far beyond my limits and helped shape me into the best version of myself. He also drove me crazy as he coached me on and off the courts and fields—with some sibling bickering sprinkled in—teaching me never to give up on myself or my dreams. He said, "If you want to be the best female tennis player in your division, you'll have to beat me first."

We spent endless hours joking, arguing, and laughing on the courts as our relationship grew into a deeper bond, a true friendship. So much of who I am is because my brother taught me by example, showing me compassion, strength, and love. He also taught me that the path of least resistance isn't always the best choice. Sometimes, you must make unpopular decisions, even in the face of others' disapproval. Throughout my life, I would talk to my brother after his passing and hear his voice of strength guide me during challenging life decisions. These life lessons he imparted to me were invaluable in all facets of my life.

When my brother was diagnosed, I couldn't jump into action fast enough. We would have done anything for each other. I assisted early on with finding doctors and treatments, even flying him to appointments for the latest treatments in other states. This was all before the internet in the late 1980s into the early 1990s. Cancer eroded his once strong foundation, eventually forcing him to live in a hospital bed, paralyzed from the waist down.

Our roles shifted as I lifted him when he was broken, and I abandoned all my responsibilities when he needed me. When I was in my second year of law school, my brother wanted to go to Magic Mountain to ride roller coasters. His body was weakening, and we could sense that soon, his ability to live life freely would be ending as the cancer would completely take over. I knew I shouldn't cut classes, with law school exams approaching. I also knew that years from then, missing classes would be far less important than missing time with my brother. I couldn't say yes fast enough.

Even though his body was in excruciating pain, cancer had stolen the vision in his right eye, and he walked with a cane some days; no one witnessing us that day in the amusement park could have known his battle would end soon. We spent the day playfully enjoying every ride like we were children, screaming at the top of our lungs on each high and low of every roller coaster while we laughed all day. Early on, I learned that choosing time and making memories was far more valuable than being responsible in certain circumstances. Time will pass, but we only get one life.

Through the years, we forged an unbreakable bond. I recall one day in the hospital, just three weeks before his passing, when he was still able to speak. I was in my last semester of law school and spent every waking moment with my brother Jeff when I wasn't studying. We were in the hospital room, and I was washing his hair and massaging his aching body. He opened his eyes between deep breaths when the nurse came in to administer pain medications, cleared his congested lungs, and proudly introduced me.

"This is my baby sister. When she was little, I took care of her; now I can't do that anymore, so she's here taking such great care of me."

He closed his eyes slowly and fell back asleep as I massaged his head and wiped away my tears. Smiling with pride and looking toward the nurse, I knew there was nowhere else in the world I would rather be.

Three weeks later, my brother passed away. He fought valiantly for twelve years as his cancer aggressively metastasized to his brain, spine, and lungs, eventually taking his life at the young age of thirty. My mind raced, and I couldn't help but feel the panic of those years he courageously battled each new diagnosis as more tumors ripped away at his athletic, healthy, young, and vibrant body.

My mind funneled down a narrow path, fearing that life again.

Would Jeff and I have to endure a similar fate? Would I have to relive that horrific nightmare and witness his suffering?

Forcing myself into the present, the words cancer and tumor were like a shockwave through my system. Denial immediately set in. Jeff was among the strongest, fittest, and healthiest people I knew; there must have been a mistake. We had plans to grow old together. Words finally made their way out, breaking the agonizing silence.

"Are you sure? We need to run more tests. I want other opinions," I demanded.

We still had to complete our future dreams together. These four short years could not be the end; we needed more time. We still had a lifetime ahead of us. I could feel myself pleading with God. *No, please, not again.* There was no way that God would be so cruel as to take two of the most influential men in my life so young, both of my Jeffs.

Waves of grief hit hard and fast. I doubled over in pain as guttural sobs spilled unabashedly from my lips. I had turned away from Jeff, but could hear his sobs and heartbreak beside me. I couldn't look into his eyes. Fear lay heavy over every part of the room as my sweaty grip clutched the sheets of the sterile bed so tightly my nails dug into my fists.

This can't be how our story ends. This can't be our truth.

I begged God for mercy.

Several agonizing minutes passed. The dark cloud of despair slowly dissipated, and we began to see a small beacon of light shining dimly through the tears. Time seemed to have stopped as my mind shifted from screams of fear, rage, and panic to survival mode. My pleading with God for mercy soon turned into making a plan of action to give us time. My thoughts shifted jaggedly from one concern to an entirely different one. Over the next several minutes, my mind wandered— from where to seek further opinions, to what our options might be, and whether this was a death sentence. Then it drifted to our families, how to break the news, and when.

Finally, Jeff and I began to talk things through. The one thing we were sure of was that calling everyone to share the horrific news was more than we could bear. We kept holding each other so we didn't fall into the dark hole of fear and shock.

Not noticing the doctors had left the room, we saw them return, waking us from our stupor. St. Jude's was an excellent local hospital, but it wasn't the type that could handle our delicate and potentially life-threatening situation. The doctors explained to us that we needed to be transferred to a larger hospital with the capabilities to acutely handle a five-centimeter tumor with teams of oncologists and surgeons. Luckily, there were more than four capable facilities within an hour's drive.

Some of the initial shock and chaos simmered to a low boil, and we began making excruciating calls to loved ones while impatiently waiting to be transferred. We started with Jeff's two children, then my two children, followed by a call to Jeff's mom. We could barely pick up the phone to make each call; speaking the words out loud was agonizing as we processed what felt like a death sentence. Pressing the send button for each call felt like an out-of-body experience—like shoveling dirt onto a casket, burying everyone's dreams in a slow-motion nightmare. Saying the word tumor out loud over and over again made our nightmare become a reality.

With each call came questions we couldn't answer. The endless sobbing, heartache, begging that it was wrong, and fear and pain in each voice, was unbearable. We couldn't stomach any more calls; hearing the fear and desperation in each voice cut deep into our souls.

We waited the next few hours to see if another hospital in our area (UCLA, USC, Cedars-Sinai, or Loma Linda) could find a bed for Jeff. Each facility was within an hour's drive from our home and well-equipped to properly diagnose and create a plan to save him.

The dreams we'd mapped out earlier that morning had abruptly turned from barbecues and travel to praying Jeff would make it to fifty. Our focus had suddenly become planning how to save Jeff's life and remove a tumor rather than getting married one day. We couldn't consider the idea that this was the end.

We learned, one by one, that none of the four hospitals could take him. We were informed that all their beds were full, and we would have to check out of the emergency room and go home to wait for a bed on Monday. I was furious.

"This is not acceptable. We are not going home," I demanded.

Continuing, I asked, "It's now Friday afternoon, and you want us to go home, lose time while the cancer is growing and killing him, and wait forty-eight hours until Monday morning to call around to see who could take him? Absolutely not, not on my watch."

From what I learned in my teens and twenties with my brother, the advocate in me came to the surface. I would not back down until someone found room for Jeff.

"We will find a hospital to see him today. Please prepare the scans so we can take them now," I said.

We left St. Jude's on a mission to find the closest and largest hospital with a campus of doctors, treatments, and options. I have no recollection of driving the forty-five minutes to Loma Linda University Hospital or what we did on the drive. We were on autopilot; so much of that day was a blur. With Jeff's medical background and my experience as a patient advocate, we believed the only way to be seen by a specialist on a Friday night was through the emergency room. As the sun set on that horrendous day, again in an emergency room, we held on, our minds racing with panic for hours as we waited for answers.

Late that night, we finally met with doctors, who performed more tests and evaluations. At the end of it all, they told us no one in oncology could see us until Saturday.

"We'll wait," I said unflinchingly.

Far past exhaustion and consumed by fear, we still needed answers and were willing to wait as long as necessary. Realizing that we had been up nearly twenty-four hours and weren't leaving, they gave us a gurney to lie on in the hallway.

We lay there that night, my petite body curled into Jeff's six-foot-long, lean frame. We spooned, holding each other tighter than ever on that thin, hard gurney with one sheet over us. The ER was full of screaming patients and loud noises, but all I remember on that darkest of nights was the sound of our intertwined hearts as we lay there, praying the sunrise would bring us answers and options.

We were jarred awake by the morning hospital shift rushing through the emergency room hallways. We slowly opened our eyes, still holding hands, as we stretched out each stiff limb and sat up. We cleared the thick, chalky taste from our mouths with gum and then went to the front desk. We checked back in, and I grabbed coffee and tea for us. Although the panic and fear were still very present, the new day, with a few hours of sleep, seemed to give us new life. We woke up eager to meet the oncologists on call that weekend, which allowed optimism to seep into our thoughts and provide us with hope.

Waiting for hours that morning, we were eventually seen by an oncologist and given a private room in the hospital. The oncologist went over the previous hospital's findings with us and then decided to perform more scans and an MRI. My parents, who lived nearby, had driven to Loma Linda to offer support and keep us company while we waited for the results. It was Saturday midday, and the room was still as the tension intensified. Few words were spoken, aside from occasional small talk meant to mask the mounting fear and desperation.

After several long hours, the door slowly opened, and a team of four doctors calmly entered the room and surrounded Jeff's bed. A heaviness came over us, and we instinctively knew the news would devastate us. We listened in horror as our worst nightmares were confirmed: It was an aggressive cancer, and Jeff had just three to six months to live.

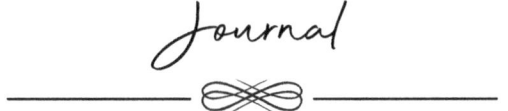

Some moments split life into "before" and "after," leaving us forever changed in an instant. Think about a time when unexpected news altered the course of your life. How did you process the first waves of shock, and what helped you find the strength to take your next step?

Chapter 7

Desperate Measures

My knees buckled, and I fell into a chair as everyone in the room began to sob and wail uncontrollably. The oxygen seemed to evaporate from the room, and I started gasping for air as I struggled to catch my breath. Jeff was lying in the bed in shock, not making a sound. My parents tried their best to console us, but there was nothing anyone could say. The diagnosis we'd received shattered our world. Only four months earlier, everything had finally aligned; the dream we had carefully crafted had just begun, and now that dream was disintegrating before our eyes.

The new reality sank in heavy and hard.

Cancer.

The word swirled ominously through my mind. Worse was the estimation of just three to six more months with my love. My heart ached—a deep, dark, crushing ache—but I couldn't just accept it.

It took a while, but once we regained our composure and could form words, we asked what our options were. There was only one, a craniotomy (a surgical procedure to remove a portion of the skull to access the brain) to remove the tumor. Jeff's eyes grew wide with terror; he knew precisely what a craniotomy entailed. Neither of us could comprehend that he had so little time left on this Earth, but to spend that time recovering from a craniotomy seemed utterly illogical. Neither of us felt that a craniotomy was a viable option.

We left the hospital that evening entirely defeated. Just forty-eight hours earlier, we were looking forward to a lifetime together. Now, we had just months. Crushed, we held each other up as we silently left the hospital and made our way home. It was our loneliest car ride.

We arrived home late Saturday night after two days of hell, in shock and dismay, and sat in the driveway, frozen from exhaustion and disbelief. Filled with trepidation, we knew that by walking inside our home, we would bring a ruthless enemy into our loving sanctuary. That destructive enemy was a part of Jeff that we had suddenly been forced to confront. We'd have to learn to coexist, but we weren't ready, so we sat silently in the car.

Drained and barely able to move, we couldn't begin to absorb what had transpired in so short a time. Since leaving home two days prior, we'd faced fear, hopelessness, rage, and complete devastation over what lay before us. Uncertain of where to begin, we sat in silence for what felt like an eternity, paralyzed by mountains of unanswered questions, which made it all too overwhelming.

We stared out the car's windshield into the still sky above as we held hands in silence. The hand-holding was unlike any other. It was a touch filled with doubt and uncertainty instead of the familiar, loving touch of comfort and adoration. The distance between us was unmistakable. Somehow, disconnecting our hearts from each other made the raw wound feel less exposed. I could feel an invisible wall between us as we sat side- by-side, not knowing what our future held or how much time was left.

Everything felt unsure. I didn't know where to begin. I didn't know what to do next. *Did we need more opinions? How much time did we have left together? Would it be three months? Could we extend it past six months?* My thoughts were filled with endless doubt. I was thinking of Jeff and what he must have felt. Panic must have been racing through his mind, knowing that his life would be cut short. My heart ached for him and the fear and pain he must have been facing in the silence.

Slowly, the emotional wall melted away, and I felt we were both ready to talk. The bone-chilling silence needed to be broken. I looked toward Jeff, avoiding eye contact, fearful if we looked into each other's eyes, I would see the horrific pain swelling up like a tidal wave and the flood of tears would start all over.

Finally, with a hollowness in my voice, I said, "Honey, let's go inside."

His handhold changed into a firm grip as if he was bracing himself. Jeff looked sharply in my direction, making eye contact as he stared deeply into my soul.

"Honeybee, I can't allow you to go through this again. No, you've lived this life before, and you don't deserve to go through this pain again. I can move back to Canada. My sisters and mom can take care of me and the cancer."

I was shocked and in disbelief that he had actually said that. Clearly, during the deafening silence, we both were thinking of very different scenarios. While he was trying to protect me from living through a life of cancer again, I was thinking of how I could save him from the cancer. Without hesitation, I sharply looked back and asked:

"If the roles were reversed, would you allow me to leave you? Would you allow someone else to lift me in my darkest hours and be my caregiver and advocate?"

An inescapable darkness hung heavy and thick as he said, "It's different if it were you, of course not. I would want to take care of you; you know I would want to be by your side. But I can't put you through this again; it's not fair to you."

"Life isn't fair; we both know that," I cried, barely controlling my volume. "It absolutely sucks sometimes, but we don't run from it! We step up and face the cards we are dealt."

By then, tears flooded my face, wet and warm, as I shakily continued.

"I love you unconditionally with every ounce of my being. This diagnosis will drastically transform our lives, but it will not end us, not without a fight. This is a battle we will fight together."

We had gone through so many hurdles to finally live the life we dreamt of together. I would not let it go that easily.

Tears streamed down Jeff's face as he said:

"How could God be so cruel? All we ever wanted was simply time together."

He wasn't wrong. It did feel incredibly cruel to allow us this gift only to test us once we received it. We had both always been very faithful in our belief in God. As admirable as Jeff's gesture was to want to protect me, we knew that was not an option.

"I just don't want to put you through all of this pain again," he said. I gently picked up his hand and reminded him that cancer wouldn't change us if we didn't let it. I could have never imagined at that moment the depths of how much that statement and our love would be tested.

We slowly took off our seatbelts with what little strength remained, feeling the immensity of the weekend. It seemed like hours had passed just sitting in the driveway when we finally summoned the energy to exit the car. As we walked through the front door of our home, it felt strangely unfamiliar and cold, filled with darkness, pain, and heavy sorrow. Nothing looked the same; it was void of light, and the warmth and joy had evaporated. We brought this unwelcome traveler, now a part of Jeff, into our home for the first time. Still wearing the same clothes, our bodies collapsed into each other as we fell onto our bed, intertwined in the fetal position. There were no more words to speak or tears to cry. We had spent the past two days unsuccessfully racing between hospitals, desperately seeking any sign of hope. There was none. Our beaten-down bodies fell hard into a deep sleep that allowed us to escape the nightmare for a handful of hours before the sun peeked in the windows.

We spent the remainder of the weekend attempting to recover and take care of the regular life responsibilities we had neglected. Amidst chaos and sorrow, we worked to prepare our lives for the next several weeks.

Monday morning, I woke to the sun shining brightly through our bedroom windows. Rising before Jeff, I slipped softly out of our bed and carefully closed the curtains we'd left open from exhaustion. I hoped he could find a few more moments of peace before waking to the nightmare we would start living. I quietly made my way downstairs, hoping to find strength in my oversized mug of dark roast.

Sitting alone at our kitchen island, I gazed at the massive ten-foot-long quartz countertop Jeff and I had picked out as we built and designed each piece of our home together. Thinking back on choosing everything from the wood flooring to the backyard pool design, every detail was selected to build the home where we would live a lifetime together. We loved the natural flow and beauty of that particular quartz. But that day, the once beautiful memory of choosing the central piece of our kitchen, where we had spent so many dinners and memories with family and friends, felt cold and empty. It was just a hard slab, empty of all movement and life. There were no more dreams for the future I could envision in our home.

In our backyard, the morning dew glistened on the spring grass as I listened to the cascading waterfalls in the pool. Jeff had set timers so I could hear them every morning with my coffee. My thoughts slipped into a harsh dose of reality as I looked around our home. I began to panic. Briefly, I saw a glimpse of the things in our home that I didn't know how to manage. They were unimportant, but my frantic mind wandered to thoughts like the waterfall timers; I didn't know how to operate them. *Would I have to ask him to show me one day soon so that I could set them on my own? What else in our home did I rely on Jeff for? What else might I have to learn to do when he was gone?*

As trivial as the thoughts felt, they reflected the idea that I would lose him and have to learn to live a life without him. A life alone, from the mundane, everyday tasks to all life's precious moments without him by my side. A sick feeling of desperation washed over me and sucked all logic from my mind. "She wished for a forever kind of love ... and she found it," my coffee mug read. Those words made my heart smile each morning, but as I sat there that day, my heart sank, thinking how my forever love would be taken from me. It felt surreal as I sat in silence alone, my body weak with shock.

I opened my phone after wiping away tears and feeling discouraged from the painful weekend. Looking through it, I noticed the date was April 30th, the twenty-third anniversary of my brother's passing.

I knew that date well but had lost track in the whirlwind of terror and shock. I took a deep breath, gently closed my eyes, and began to talk to my brother Jeff while tears poured violently out of my already emotionally drained body. God, I missed my brother; his support, comfort, and insight were invaluable growing up. At twenty-six, I had experienced living with years of a life-threatening illness, treatments, and his eventual passing at the age of thirty. My brother was the central person in my youth. We'd been inseparable, and he had helped shape my foundation; losing him was monumental.

That morning, somewhere between sobbing and feeling sorry for myself and thinking of both my Jeffs, I began to scour through my phone to review what transpired over that long weekend of diagnosis and despair that left us shattered. With the caffeine starting to kick in and more conversations with my brother, I found myself retrieving my faith in God. I spent time in solace and prayer that morning, looking for guidance. My adrenaline eventually kicked into high gear, and the fear of losing Jeff took over. I felt my body shift from wallowing in pity to preparing for action. I knew we had to come up with a plan. There was so much to be done, and I needed to move quickly. Although I wanted to sit in self-pity, I knew I couldn't; there was no time to waste.

Pulling out my computer, I researched the diagnosis, the type of cancer, and any doctors or hospitals specializing in that field who could save Jeff or at least buy him time. At that moment, on the anniversary of my brother's passing, I found gratitude. I was reminded and so very grateful for the tools now available at our fingertips, unlike when my brother was diagnosed in the 1980s. That realization provoked unwanted thoughts, recalling the torturous treatments and emotional trauma that we endured during the twelve years spent trying to save my brother Jeff before ultimately losing him in 1995. I could feel myself starting to peel back the deep layers of scars on my heart where I stored those memories of my brother and his battle. That morning, however, was not the time for reflective sorrow. I needed to temporarily cover that deep and painful scar so I could focus forward to execute a strategy to save my love, Jeff.

I researched everything I could find on the squamous cell sinus cancer that was delicately intertwining itself on Jeff's optic nerve at the skull base. I felt sure there must be more advanced surgeries or options that wouldn't involve opening up Jeff's skull with a craniotomy, which meant a lengthy recuperation that would expose him to complications. This extensive recovery would also limit his options for immediate additional treatments, limiting his chance to increase his survival past the three to six-month prognosis. I had nothing to go on but hope and faith.

As I scrolled through the texts and Google searches on my phone, it revealed who I had communicated with over the past few days. Everything had been a giant blur of intense panic and chaos from the overwhelming fear. I was surprised to find that I had searched for answers and various resources during the horrific weekend ordeal. In my desperation over the weekend, I had messaged dozens of my contacts to see if they knew anyone who had any experience with sinus surgery and skull base tumors. Maybe someone knew someone who had gone through an experience that could assist my research. It was a long shot that paid off. One of the names I heard from two friends was Dr. Jeffrey Suh.

In all my messaging with my network of friends across the country, two friends mentioned a doctor they had heard of at UCLA, Dr. Suh, who specializes in surgeries in the sinus region. Our dear friends Heather and Ryan knew someone who had gone to Dr. Suh to remove polyps and highly recommended him for sinus surgery. Then, in another text, other dear friends, Stephanie and Doug, recommended Dr. Suh for sinus surgery through one of Doug's friends, who had also been a patient.

I found Dr. Suh's bio online and read about his expertise. At the time, Dr. Suh was one of five surgeons in the U.S. in his field of head, neck, and skull base surgeries, and he performed a surgery that

I believed might be suitable for Jeff. He was trained in endoscopic cranial base surgery and the management of sinus and skull base tumors. Everything was pointing in the direction of Dr. Suh.

It was Monday morning, and I wanted to be the first call when they opened at 8:00 a.m. At precisely 7:59 a.m., I called Dr. Suh's office at UCLA, unsure exactly what I was asking for when his assistant, Antonio, answered. Still feeling vulnerable, I fought back tears with a long pause as I felt a lump rise in my throat, making it difficult to speak. Finally, I was able to get the words out with panic and urgency.

"My fiancé has an aggressive cancer, and you may be our only hope. We've been at different hospitals all weekend, and after doing some research, I think Dr. Suh can help us."

The kind voice on the other end gently explained, "I'm so sorry to hear this. However, we are booked for weeks; we can set you up with an appointment at the end of May."

I desperately stated, "You don't understand." I persistently continued, "The other doctors want to operate and do a craniotomy immediately. We've spent the weekend at hospitals and ERs, and we don't have four weeks to wait; he was given a few months to live."

Again, Antonio explained how sorry he was, but that they were booked solid.

I tried to explain our situation calmly, but I needed them to feel the desperation and panic simmering frantically inside me. This was life and death; they needed to understand that fast.

"You're our only hope. They want to cut open his skull and perform a craniotomy with little to no chance of prolonging the diagnosis of three to six months, leaving Jeff with an extensive and complicated recovery for his final days. From everything I've heard and read, Dr. Suh may be able to help my fiancé and possibly save his life."

Again, I urgently pleaded, "Please, can you please look for any time? We will be there whenever you tell us to!"

Antonio was calm and patient as he listened, then put me on hold. I waited with a sick feeling in my gut, aware we had no other options. I began to pray to God. The on-hold music oddly calmed my nerves, which I needed. It felt as if the cancer inside Jeff was growing and spreading exponentially by the minute. When I heard the phone click back, I held my breath.

"Can you bring Jeff in today?" Antonio asked me.

"Absolutely!" I cried out eagerly, thanking him.

He explained there were no openings that day, but if we were willing to sit in the waiting room, we could come to the office and see if Dr. Suh could find a few moments to see Jeff. I couldn't thank him enough and told him I would wake up Jeff, and we'd leave immediately.

As I crept upstairs, I wanted to shout out, "Honey, I've got great news!" But was it? I didn't know what Dr. Suh's diagnosis or possible surgery option would be. For all I knew, we might arrive home that night in the same position. I had no idea; I just knew we had to try. I softly crawled back under the sheets and into bed next to Jeff to slowly wake him into our new reality.

Caressing his back, I optimistically said, "Honey, I know how thoroughly exhausted you are, but can you get dressed?"

Eyes barely opening, he gently asked, "Why?"

I explained to him that we needed to drive to UCLA to see a specialist and then described what had developed that morning. He could barely speak with fear and fatigue plaguing him. "Okay, Honeybee. If you think we should go, then I'll get dressed."

I didn't want to overstate what the appointment may or may not be. I honestly had no idea, but my instincts knew the only option we had been given over the weekend was not worth considering yet. We needed to uncover every possible option aggressively, and it had to be done within days to beat the clock on the impending craniotomy surgery. I explained that it would be a long wait and that we should bring water and snacks, but I couldn't bring myself to tell him that we might not actually see Dr. Suh.

On the drive to the Ronald Reagan UCLA Medical Center, the car was filled with silence and sadness that consumed us. I was trying to hold back all feelings of hope. I needed to protect myself and Jeff. No directions were needed, as I knew that drive like the back of my hand; it was not only my alma mater but also where my brother Jeff received treatments in the early 1990s. There were so many parallels I couldn't pretend they didn't exist. But I couldn't let those thoughts creep in, wondering if the journey and outcome would be the same. I needed to lay that twenty-three-year-old scar to rest so I could focus on the battle ahead. I nudged myself back into the present. In that moment, we were focused on saving and extending a life, not remembering one.

Jeff and I sat patiently for hours in Dr. Suh's office. After a long wait, we were called back, our hearts racing with optimism and fear that we would be left with the same disheartening news. A few minutes later, the tall and friendly doctor walked in with a calming demeanor. His credentials didn't match his youthful appearance.

He squeezed us between his patients, yet Dr. Suh seemed in no hurry. Instead, his calm and compassionate nature brought a much-needed tranquility to the room. We were intrigued by how time seemed not to exist as Dr. Suh patiently extended his time and knowledge, answering our many questions. He reviewed his medical records and the scans we brought, performed some tests, and examined Jeff.

Once finished, Dr. Suh looked at us and stated with certainty, "I can take care of this. I will enter through Jeff's nasal passage endoscopically and remove the majority of the tumor with minimal side effects and a very short recovery."

Stunned, we both began to cry as relief washed over us, and smiles slowly erased the panic etched on our faces. The news felt impossible and surreal. For the first time in days, we could breathe.

"Really, you can remove this large mass with no craniotomy?" I asked.

He affirmed. We felt tremendously grateful and hopeful, filled with a new sense of optimism. The news was beyond encouraging; we were positively ecstatic. It was exactly what we were looking for. In seventy-two hours, we had gone from three to six months to live ... to hope.

It would be a minimally invasive surgery that could remove most of Jeff's tumor—a hopeful alternative and a stark contrast to the intensity of a full craniotomy. There were reduced side effects, no scarring, no cutting his skull or brain open, and he would be back home in a few days with no long recovery. Dr. Suh explained that by using an endoscope to delicately enter Jeff's nasal passage, he could remove most of the five-centimeter tumor in the front section of the skull base, all while avoiding healthy tissue and doing everything he could to try and preserve his vision.

Once our heightened emotions and relief subsided, they gave way to more questions.

"When would this all happen?" I asked.

"We can take care of this next week," Dr. Suh stated nonchalantly. *Is he serious? I thought. How could he remove the tumor next week?* I began crying tears of joy again as I witnessed the relief on Jeff's face as his demeanor shifted. I could see his shoulders release as an enormous breath was exhaled, and his eyes widened. Dr. Suh patiently gave us the time and space we needed.

My heart was pounding out of my chest with excitement as we held each other. I could feel the immense heaviness lift from Jeff as well. One moment, we were lost, and in the next breath, we felt safe and secure. We knew it was just the beginning of our battle, but we had so much to fight for. We were happy to have a starting point, something we could embrace and hold onto tightly, a life jacket of tangible hope. Heightened emotions surged through our veins as we held each other. I felt like all our plans for a future together would still have the possibility of survival. I knew it was up to us to find the courage to enter the battle we faced with an armor made of love and strength.

Jeff and I couldn't wait to call the kids, Jeff's mom, and all the family on our drive home. We knew they, too, had been living the same nightmare from afar for the past few days. We relished hearing each one of their voices as we shared the fantastic news that hope had been found. Each voice was elated with joy, the complete opposite of the calls we'd made on Friday. We had a newfound energy that gave us the strength to forge forward.

We made our way back into Chino Hills, stopping for a celebratory dinner. That's when I shared something with Jeff that I had been holding inside all day.

Sitting beside each other, I held his hand and asked, "Honey, do you know what today is?"

There had been so much swirling around us the past few days that I didn't expect him to remember that it was the twenty-third anniversary of my brother's passing, so I reminded him. I had held my breath all day, thinking it might be another day of despair, just like in 1995. Instead, that day, we celebrated the first of many victories we would steadfastly fight for over the years.

Jeff and I were resolved to fight for time together. I proclaimed, "Honey, from now on, April 30th will always be a reminder of hope, not heartache."

During the dozens of medical challenges we would face in the years to come, we would remind ourselves of our victory that day. We had built a strong foundation of mutual respect, trust, and a deep connection, creating a formidable bond that would allow our love to overcome seemingly insurmountable trials.

That four-day nightmare taught us that we would never let a diagnosis dictate our destiny or infect our love.

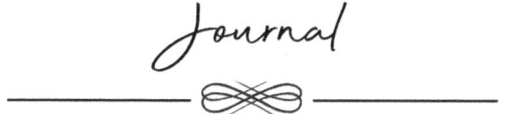

Sometimes hope appears in the unlikeliest moments, just when you've been told to give up. Write about a time when you were faced with a situation that seemed impossible, yet you chose to push forward. What gave you the courage to defy the odds, and how did that decision shape what came next?

Chapter 8

SUMMER AFTER THE DIAGNOSIS

After receiving the news that Dr. Suh could remove most of the tumor, our marathon of endless miles began. Once again, we needed to be all in to give Jeff and our future together the best possible odds. Our resolve to buy more time and our unwavering dedication to each other would be challenged relentlessly. There was no way to prepare for the battle we faced; it would test us in every way—emotionally, mentally, and physically. Above all, it would test our love.

We prayed for a chance to fight, and Dr. Suh had given us that. The surgery gave us a chance to continue to dream of a lifetime together. On Thursday, May 3, 2018, we met with Dr. Suh for a pre-op to review everything we should expect for the procedure the following Monday. The emotions were turbulent; a layer of anxiety hung over us like a thick blanket. We were hopeful yet tense, knowing the operation drew near. Everything was ready.

The weekend before the surgery, we drove to one of our favorite places to find solace and quiet time alone: the beach at sunset. We were preparing for and willing to take on a long fight, far beyond three to six months. We knew the longer the fight was, the more time we would have for our future. We believed that if we had a chance for time, it would be a lengthy battle filled with treatments and surgeries, long days, and grueling nights. We wanted time alone to be our "old" selves before the surgery and the effects of cancer in all its vicious wrath began on Monday. We had no idea what the future held, so we took that opportunity to enjoy our last few moments before the battle began. We went to our favorite place, the Surf and Sand in Laguna Beach, a spot filled with beautiful memories.

That night, as we watched the sunset, Jeff leaned into me, saying, "There will never be a sunset without you, Honeybee." I was breathless with the loving and delicate emotions he conveyed. But suddenly, I was struck with despair as I realized he didn't say I would never have a sunset without him. Deep inside, we both knew the harsh reality of what we were up against, but we couldn't say it out loud. Rather than fear the unknowns we would soon face, we compelled ourselves to focus on what was certain at that moment: the promise of tomorrow.

Despite the terror of our future weighing heavily, we found ways to escape those ever-present thoughts. We enjoyed the coastline's natural beauty and the vibrant sunset as we breathed in fresh ocean air and held each other tightly. We made a conscious effort not to discuss the upcoming surgery or Jeff's cancer. Instead, we cherished the peaceful moments. We allowed ourselves to drift into a soft focus and dream far away from reality and into romanticism, giving ourselves a reprieve from what lay just around the corner.

Over dinner, we grabbed a napkin and made a bucket list of everything we still wanted to experience together. We dreamt of experiences we hadn't had yet, including some local road trip getaways. Jeff had never driven up the California coastline to see Big Sur, the Redwood trees, and the infamous Pebble Beach golf course along the seventeen-mile drive. It was his dream to play at Pebble Beach. Jeff also wanted to experience some new parts of Europe and travel to the Caribbean to experience the warm, turquoise, crystal-clear waters. High on the list was watching his favorite football team, the Seattle Seahawks, play in their home stadium.

We snuggled into each other, our hearts filled with romantic dreams and anxious uncertainty as we mapped out a future of hope on a cocktail napkin. We prayed that God would show mercy on us so we could check each one off the list. It wasn't the traveling that was vital; instead, each check would signify we were winning the battle against time. Each item checked off the list would give us hope and reinforce the triumph of knowing we beat the three-to-six-month diagnosis.

That night, we threw practicality into the ocean, never wondering if or how we could accomplish our goals. Instead, we let our thoughts swim in dreams for the future. We knew the list was lofty, but as the months relentlessly went on and the cancer took its toll, that list of dreams helped keep our spirits high. We continually peeked at that list as a way to escape, and it gave us a brighter future to look forward to at the end of each battle.

We were equally anxious and excited for the delicate and lengthy surgery Dr. Suh would perform to remove the cancer. The unwelcome traveler in Jeff's body brought with it profound anxiety. The five-centimeter tumor was a part of Jeff that we despised, but it was a part of him. The surgery couldn't arrive fast enough. Jeff's children and my two children flew into town, along with my dear friend Heather from Boise, Idaho.

May 7, 2018, signified hope. It brought with it the promise of more time to love each other, more time for Jeff to spend with family and friends, and maybe enough time for a cure or new treatment to be discovered. We looked at each day after as a gift and a blessing. Admittedly, we were selfish. We wanted as many gifts as God would bestow upon us. Faithfully, we were willing to do all the work put before us each day. We didn't know how to give up. We only knew how to stay strong in our convictions and faiths and believed that if we showed up, God would create a path for us to forge forward. It was a glorious and grueling road God paved for us, but not all roads lead to answered prayers. All we could do was control our own choices along the way and hope for the best.

The morning of the surgery, the silence in the car was deafening as we drove to UCLA with our bags packed. We would spend a few days there as Jeff recovered from his operation. My mind was a roller coaster of emotions; I tried to control the throttle and maintain my composure at a steady pace, somewhere between the peaks and valleys. Judging by the stiffness of Jeff's movements and his hundred-yard stare, I could tell he was doing the same. Our nerves were on high alert. We held hands while the doctors, nurses, and anesthesiologists worked diligently to prepare for the complicated and highly specialized surgery.

Sitting alone, waiting for Jeff to be taken to the operating room, I told him, "Honey, we've got this. I will be right here when you come out of surgery, and we will do everything in our power to win this battle and buy as much time as possible. I will never give up hope." Jeff looked at me. "Honeybee, I couldn't love you more. You are my everything." I held tightly onto his hands. Moments later, the nurses entered the room and began wheeling him down the long hall. I walked next to his gurney with all his IVs and drips hanging beside him for as long as they would let me before he was taken behind the big, white double doors. Our pinkies interlocked as we softly kissed goodbye before disconnecting as he was wheeled away. My heart thundered like a stampede in my chest as Jeff disappeared through two large, ominous doors at the end of the stark white hall.

Left alone in the cold, desolate corridors, I collapsed against a wall, sobbing as I slid to the floor. There, I prayed God would guide Dr. Suh's skilled hands to carefully remove the tumor wrapped around the sensitive optic nerves that it was threatening. We knew there was a strong possibility that Jeff could lose vision in his right eye. As the fear began to take over, I forced myself to lean on faith and the wonderful circle of support inside and outside of the hospital.

When I could collect myself, I walked out to the waiting room, which was surrounded by large windows, soft chairs, and a tranquil garden. There, I found my parents, Heather, and all the kids congregating in a large space. They had come to the hospital so we could all support each other. Leaving the stark white hallway, I was relieved to walk into a room filled with love. Tension hung thick and heavy over everyone gathered, making conversation difficult and awkward. We'd all been sitting in uncomfortable silence when my dad offered to go to the cafeteria and see what he could find.

Walking back into the waiting area filled with friends and strangers, he broke the uncomfortable silence by exclaiming loudly, "Does anyone want a soft serve cone?"

My dad, a larger-than-life, loveable personality, was always unapologetically himself, which we all adored as it brought warmth and familiarity into the waiting room. Soon, my parents returned with ice cream cones for everyone; it was a welcome distraction. Eating in silence, the room heavy with stillness—until my dad's voice rang out, just below a shout, cutting through the quiet like a crack of thunder.

"Ah shit Barb, can you believe this? I spilled ice cream on my favorite shirt."

Everyone in the room looked at my dad and instantly laughed. The tension quickly melted away like the ice cream on his cone.

A few hours later, the anxiety in the room skyrocketed when Dr. Suh walked calmly through the waiting room doors. My body immediately tensed, my stomach twisted tight, and I became hot and sweaty as my stress level peaked. I tried to read his face as he approached, looking for any signs, anything positive, but I couldn't get a read.

Taking a deep breath, I tried to compose myself as Dr. Suh stopped before me.

"It was a successful surgery, and Jeff's doing well in recovery." Focused on communicating the facts of Jeff's outcome, he continued, "We were able to get eighty percent of the tumor that was impinging on his optic nerve at the base of his skull. Considering the size and location of the tumor, eighty percent was what we expected and hoped for."

A wave of relief rushed over me, but there was a central question I needed answered before I could breathe again.

Fearing the answer, I nervously asked, "Dr. Suh, were you able to save his vision?" I braced myself for the answer.

"Yes," he confidently stated.

I let out a deep sigh of relief and was overwhelmed with a flood of tears. We expressed our deepest gratitude to Dr. Suh for making the surgery possible. We greatly appreciated the new lease on life he had given Jeff. I went out to the garden with Heather and continued crying. I was grateful but also afraid of the unknown twenty percent battle that remained. We knew that soon phase two would begin; the tumor was eighty percent gone, but an aggressive cancer remained. We had no idea how many phases were ahead of us.

Jeff and I were left alone in the room once everyone had had a chance to visit him. That evening, I pulled up the chair in his room and made the first of dozens of beds with a hospital sheet, my pillow, and the warm hospital blankets from the warming machine. I was inordinately exhausted from the onslaught of overwhelming emotions I'd lived through that week. Believing Jeff's life might soon be over, then finding hope that he might have more time, perhaps even the possibility of survival—it was all too much to process in so short a time. We held hands, lying in separate beds next to each other. I quietly thanked God for guiding us during the ten days following Jeff's diagnosis as we peacefully drifted off to sleep awash in new hope.

The surgery had been minimally invasive, so Jeff was only in the hospital for a few days to recover and be observed. The surgery was the first step. The next step was to design an attack strategy for the remaining twenty percent of the tumor. Time was of the greatest essence. The extremely aggressive cancer was metastasizing (spreading). Although there was no way to detect how quickly it would spread, based on the doctor's projections, we feared we couldn't keep up with the rate at which the cancer might travel to other parts of his body. The doctors concluded that the cancer may soon spread to his brain, a battle we would face if and when it was detected. But to start, the worry and focus were clear and concise: stop the spread of the cancer, and attack and destroy what we already knew was present. We couldn't allow ourselves to speculate on what we couldn't control.

I didn't want to waste one moment. Before we left UCLA Hospital, following the three-day post-op stay, I worked to set up several appointments with different hospitals to discuss Jeff's treatment options. Once home, we spent a few days recovering, then got right back to looking into all our options as we attended appointments at hospitals throughout the area, which felt more like interviews. Each appointment helped us determine if it was the right facility for us.

At one appointment, we sat in a tiny, cold clinician's room where we clung to each other, hoping someone could offer a miracle to save him. Jeff's life was in the hands of each professional we met with. We felt exposed and more vulnerable than ever as we sought comfort, solutions, and candor. After reviewing Jeff's records and examining him, the doctor walked into the room and said there was little hope for Jeff to live past the end of that year. Having just come out of a surgery that brought us hope, the doctor's callous assessment knocked the wind out of us. That was not our doctor.

We didn't want anyone to sugarcoat things; we didn't need kid gloves. For us, even if there was little hope that Jeff would live past the end of the year, we wanted a team that would focus on the small hope of survival beyond that, not the death sentence. It was crucial that we received honesty and compassion from a team of doctors willing to take on a fight with us. We needed to know what we were fighting and who would fight with us. Even though the doctor's words were disheartening, somehow, we heard the word "hope." It wasn't much, but it was hope, and we realized that's all we needed.

In our minds, we were already ahead of the game. We gave Jeff the best start possible by forgoing the craniotomy for a less invasive option. That choice meant his body was immediately ready to handle radiation and chemotherapy (chemo) to rid him of the remaining twenty percent. Jeff could go into the next phase from a position of strength rather than being weakened and going through a long recovery. This was essential as it expanded our options and expedited our timeframe.

Following calls and appointments with numerous doctors, we quickly determined Loma Linda was our most effective option, with the most aggressive approach. Fortunately, Loma Linda was only forty-five minutes from our home (without Southern California traffic), making the commute relatively easy. We lived in a region surrounded by some of the world's most skilled doctors and institutions. We were lucky to have many outstanding choices. With advanced medicines and treatments surrounding us, combined with our determination and tenacity, Jeff and I knew that we could put up one hell of a fight.

We were determined to make sure cancer did not overwhelm our hearts so we wouldn't lose each other in the fight; it wasn't always easy. We would be forced to navigate countless struggles in our relationship over the next three years. But we were dedicated to fighting this unwelcome traveler and maintaining the love we had fought so hard for. We quickly learned our mindset had to be stronger than the anguish. We decided early on that the initial diagnosis would not dictate our destiny or infect our love.

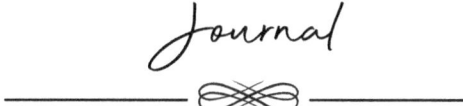

Hope can live alongside fear, and sometimes they hold hands while you walk into the unknown. Think about a time when you balanced excitement for the future with the weight of uncertainty. How did you keep your spirit from breaking, and what gave you the strength to keep dreaming?

Chapter 9
THE PLAN

The beginning of summer 2018 found us at Loma Linda for an appointment. They offered Jeff the radiation and chemo options, and we didn't need any time to answer.

Few words were spoken between us before Jeff said, "If we have any shot at beating this, or at least buying more time, we have to use the most aggressive treatments available." I agreed.

Dr. Suh gave us the best possible start. Now, we were in the hands of Loma Linda University Cancer Center, the world's first hospital-based proton therapy facility. The proton therapy they offered was an advanced type of radiation therapy that directly targets a tumor with precise treatment doses and fewer side effects. We began mapping out a plan with the radiation oncology team, which took weeks to design.

The focus of the radiation team was to target and attack the tumors with proton therapy precision that directly aimed at designated marks on Jeff's head, neck, and skull base with laser beams coming from numerous angles. We chose a very aggressive radiation therapy plan; our goal was to eradicate as much of the cancer in Jeff's body as we could without destroying him in the process. The extreme approach would last eight weeks straight, starting the first week of June and ending the last week of July, leaving Jeff with only Saturdays and Sundays to rest.

The technician who walked Jeff in and out of the radiation stated that in all the years he had worked with the proton radiation machine, he had never seen one person endure as much radiation as Jeff. The statement reassured us that we were aggressive in our approach, thereby giving him the best odds. It also scared the hell out of us, knowing the unbearable torture we chose to put Jeff's body through.

Once we decided on our radiation strategy, we went over to the chemo department. The doctors explained the various options available for Jeff, offering us three different forms of chemo treatments, each varying in strength and the length of time they are administered. Two of the options would take a less aggressive approach. Those options provided less potency and would be spread intermittently over many months, which meant he would endure fewer side effects. The third option, cisplatin, is what we chose. It was the most aggressive option that included a grueling eight-week continuous schedule alongside the radiation. They explained all the risks of taking on this extremely aggressive chemo approach, administered simultaneously with our already aggressive proton radiation plan.

Jeff and I knew that we were committed to doing anything in our power to save his life, including taking Jeff's body to the brink of death with the hope of bringing him back to life cancer-free. If it didn't work, we hoped it would buy us enough time to get to the next scan and check another dream off our bucket list. Even with the detailed and intense plan, there were no guarantees that we wouldn't end up in the same three-to-six-month position afterward. Despite it all, we were willing to take the risk.

I knew my role as advocate and caregiver would be overwhelming, and that Jeff's body would be tortured. We weren't naive about the nightmare we were soon to encounter. We needed to mentally prepare ourselves the best we could for what lay ahead. We weren't looking for a band-aid but a cure, or at least a chance to buy more time.

We knew that summer would be a living hell, but we were both fully committed. There was no indecisiveness; we knew what needed to be done. Our resolution was strong, and our love was stronger. We made up our minds and had the next couple of weeks to get our personal lives in order so we could devote all our energy and focus on Jeff's treatments. I needed to be decisive in everything from that moment forward.

His body would be beaten down to the point he would want to give up or die, and I would need to bravely support and encourage him to find the courage to fight when there was nothing left to give. I knew our love would be tested, and our resolve to cohesively tighten our bond would be crucial. The radiation and chemo would provide the medication to kill the cancer, but Jeff's body and soul would need nurturing on the days his will to fight was depleted. I'd be his center of support, lead decision-maker, and place of comfort and reassurance.

We sat in the hospital administrator's office, ready to sign the final paperwork for Jeff's treatments. But before we could sign them, the Loma Linda Hospital administrator called the insurance company to discuss a discrepancy in how the payments would be made. Our insurance had an issue regarding whether the aggressive and extensive approach we chose was necessary. The insurance company asked us to hold off on the treatments until they could determine the necessity of such an extreme treatment plan. The discussion went on for a while and turned into a heated debate. There was no time to lose. We believed we'd come up with the most effective plan to give Jeff the best odds of beating the cancer. Confident in our choices, we did not feel it necessary to waste valuable time discussing it further.

After a lengthy argument with the insurance company, I saw that nothing would be resolved. So, I declared, "That's enough. We're doing this unless you devise a better plan immediately. Otherwise, this is the plan. You're focused on costs, and I'm focused on saving his life. We are at an impasse."

At a very early age, I learned from my dad, a decisive poker player, that if you know your hand, play it with conviction. Don't second-guess yourself, and don't back down. That was one of those moments. I was ready to play poker, and I called their bluff. It was not a game for us; it was Jeff's life. It was non-negotiable. He needed the treatments without delay to give him the best chance for survival.

Hanging up the phone, I looked over at the hospital administrator and asked her the cash price. She looked at me like I had three heads.

"Uh, ma'am, you realize this is going to be a huge bill with the extensive radiation and chemo plan they are prescribing for Jeff? Are you sure you want to do this?"

Without hesitation, I firmly stated, "I am absolutely certain. I know the amount will be enormous; I need you to give me that number."

Once I was given the dollar amount, I grabbed my wallet and pulled out all three credit cards. That day, in the Loma Linda administrator's office, I asked them to wait patiently while I made some calls. I picked up my phone and dialed the first of three numbers. Each call was the same as the first.

"Hi, my fiancé was diagnosed with an aggressive cancer, and he needs treatment immediately. I need to increase my limit. How much can you give me?"

If the amount wasn't enough, I asked them to look at my credit history and excellent credit scores and again asked for a higher amount, which required a supervisor to approve the significant increase. I hung up with the last credit card and laid each one in front of the administrator with the exact amounts she should put on each credit card. She was stunned by what had transpired. Together, it totaled over $75,000.

In my mind, there was no time to mess around; we couldn't waste one day. Every hour delayed would mean the cancer was gaining the upper hand. We were moving forward fast. The train was in motion, and the insurance company could either get on board or not, but we were leaving the station. I knew the fight wasn't over with the insurance company, but I also knew the fight to save Jeff preempted the battle over who would pay the bill.

Ultimately, the fight with the insurance company would last another eight weeks, the length of Jeff's treatments. We sat and watched as each card was maxed out for the radiation and chemo treatments. Though it was terrifying, I was exceedingly grateful to have that option. I know not everyone does. I had laser focus, no different than the proton radiation, and we both had one job that summer: to save Jeff's life.

With three kids in college, a mortgage payment, medical bills, and all the other regular expenses, I wasn't made of steel. The strain of so much added debt scared the hell out of me. But financial worries at that moment were nothing compared to losing Jeff. Once again, I couldn't let fear get in the way of what I knew I needed to do. That became a pattern and the anthem for our relationship. Jeff and I had a lifetime to share, and I was determined to do everything in my power to increase our odds.

To survive the summer intact, I'd need to map out my strategy. Thankfully, we had a circle of especially supportive family and friends. I mapped out each week where I would need help at our business or with Jeff. He needed to be driven five days a week, two hours round-trip, for treatment. On top of the drive, waiting at the hospital lasted three to five hours. Following each treatment, Jeff needed to be tended to once he arrived home so he could recover and prepare to do it again the next day. Although work was not the top priority, medical and personal bills were beginning to accumulate, and our business was less than six months old. We needed it to survive the grueling summer as well.

Throughout those eight weeks of treatment, Jeff's family flew in from Canada to assist with our many needs. My children and family also stepped up with the driving schedule and helped at our home. Our friends were readily available, and we had no lack of loving support—they helped with groceries, meals, and driving, and provided shoulders to lean on. One of our great sources of support that summer was my dear friend Stephanie from New York, who flew in for two weeks to help drive Jeff to his treatments and go into our business so I could be with Jeff.

The first few weeks of treatments went relatively smoothly for Jeff, who had only slight nausea and fatigue. We knew the side effects wouldn't present themselves immediately, but it was only a matter of time before the consequences of the battle would find us; there was no escaping the inevitable. We braced for the monsters infiltrating Jeff's body to rear their ugly heads.

By mid-summer, the collateral damage of radiation and chemo began to take hold of his body. He was being destroyed from the inside out in a desperate effort to save him, to save us. He barely had time to recover from each round of chemo and radiation before he was at it again the next day. It was a grueling five-day-a-week schedule that beat relentlessly on his continually diminishing frame. By the end of the eight weeks, he could barely walk into his appointments, finally giving in to being pushed in a wheelchair.

Intentionally choosing that path felt cruel at times as I watched the torture continue. Many days, remorse crept in. It was then that I forced my subconscious to take a back seat, willing my conscience to lead the way to hope. It was necessary to mentally push away all thoughts of guilt and emotions to complete the agonizing treatments. If we had allowed our feelings to control medical decisions, neither of us would have ever agreed to subject him to so much anguish.

Initially, we were most concerned with chemo and the side effects it would cause. We hadn't expected the radiation to cause so much collateral damage to his body. Combining the two simultaneously proved too much on some days. We expected fatigue and exhaustion from the radiation, but were not prepared for the development of severe burns.

During Jeff's forty days of radiation, we would take a special elevator to the basement level of the hospital, where natural light was blocked out. Each day, I walked Jeff down the long corridor and into the radiation room where his kind and compassionate technicians awaited. The room housing the massive proton machine appeared to be two stories tall, enormous in stature and width. Unlike other radiation machines I had seen, which resembled MRI machines in standard-sized rooms, the magnitude of the room that stored the proton radiation therapy machine was immense, and everything regarding the machine was different.

The enormity of the room and the massive walls surrounding us were incredibly intimidating. Once Jeff was on the bed, a push of a button automatically guided the bed over a hollow bay, where he would appear suspended in the air, all within the confines of a vast, open capsule. It was ominous. It resembled the vortex you ride into on the Space Mountain ride at Disneyland.

Days before treatments started, a specialized mask was created specifically for Jeff, which took close to an hour to make while he lay perfectly still. The mask was constructed by initially warming plastic to become soft and pliable. Then, it was placed over his face so it would contour perfectly to fit him before being allowed to cool and harden. Once the mask was constructed and formed to his head, as it hardened, it remained tough and solidified, not losing shape.

The technicians placed the custom-designed mask to form perfectly over his neck and head before each treatment. The plastic material had tiny, pin-sized holes over its entirety so he could breathe as they snuggly fit it onto his face. The mask confined him as he lay still on a hard, flat radiation table. Each mask could be used for the intended treatments but not for future treatments; another mask would need to be designed for each radiation treatment plan thereafter.

As Jeff lay on the long, cold table each day, they would cover him in warm blankets since his body was usually well below normal temperature. Before every treatment, we would grab pinkies, and I would give my love a soft kiss before the mask was firmly fitted onto his head and down to his collarbone. Then we said a quiet prayer that God would guide the proton radiation to destroy the tumors. The team would tighten screws on the side of the mask into the sides of his skull. The indentations from the screws were visible for hours following the procedure. They slowly smoothed out and were gone by the time we arrived home later.

Only in the dark and quiet hours late at night would he occasionally share with me the claustrophobia and fear those masks and machines unleashed upon him and how they tormented his thoughts. Each treatment left him with deeply rooted emotional scars.

Seeing him in the archaic-looking contraption that hid his piercing baby blues never got easy. I held back my tears each time I left him alone in the radiation room. Only once I was out of the room would I slowly let the tears stream down my cheeks. Through it all, I knew my emotional pain was inconsequential compared to the extreme suffering Jeff was enduring. Each radiation session lasted two to three hours and took its toll as they stacked upon each other every day, significantly diminishing his ability to recover as the days progressed.

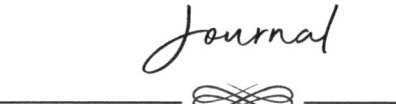

Sometimes the most courageous choice is the one that pushes you, and those you love, to the very edge. Think of a time when you had to commit fully to a difficult decision, knowing the road ahead would be grueling. What gave you the conviction to move forward, and how did you reconcile the risks with the hope for the outcome?

Chapter 10
SUMMER OF HELL

The smell of barbecues and the joy of summer travels were well underway. Meanwhile, we spent our days in anguish deep in hospital basements as we focused on Jeff's daily treatments. By the Fourth of July, Southern California's temperatures were well into the high nineties, and even hotter in Loma Linda, located further east and closer to the desert. The radiation continuously pierced and scorched Jeff's skin, turning it into a dark red and eventually a deep purple that hardened and blistered.

The radiation continued to blaze through layers of skin to find its way to the tumors, burning and searing every inch of his neck and face. With the intense summer heat, the burns on his already fragile and injured head were made more unbearable. Jeff's skin had become cruelly sensitive to the heat. To keep him out of the sun, we kept him covered in the car, and I made sure we dropped him off at the hospital's front entrance in the shade so the sun couldn't do any further damage to his exposed raw layers of tender skin.

Routine tasks like taking a shower or lying in bed became brutal activities. Shower water felt like sharp knives cutting into raw wounds on his skin. The skin on his face, head, neck, and ears peeled and ripped away as he lifted off of the bed sheets with each movement. At night, I carefully applied a salve to treat his second- and third-degree burns. I could feel the stickiness of the salve on my fingers, gripping onto his raw burn wounds as he held back screams of pain with each touch of my finger. Every dab onto the raw surface broke my heart into pieces, knowing we voluntarily chose that course of action. Jeff's bravery during those times gave me the strength and fortitude to push forward.

Following each radiation treatment, I met Jeff in the hallway and helped guide him over to the chemo section of the hospital. The chemo area had a couple dozen soft lounge chairs for patients to comfortably rest while drugs were administered through an IV drip. The chemo side effects soon hit full force, and Jeff's appetite became nonexistent.

The chemo was every other day for a few hours, either before or after the radiation. Cancer cells grow and multiply much quicker than other cells in the body, and the chemo was intended to kill the fast-growing cells. However, chemo does not target a specific area like radiation does. Instead, chemo works throughout one's body, attacking all the cells. The chemo drug, unlike radiation, cannot discern between healthy and cancerous cells, and it cannot choose which cells to attack, so it eradicates all cells in its path. Side effects were inevitable. Numerous types of chemo vary in intensity and length of treatment, which is reflected in the side effects. But because we chose such an aggressive approach, Jeff's body was pushed to extreme limits. Some days, it seemed as though we brought him to the very edge of death.

He developed extremely sensitive and painful mouth sores, a direct result of both the chemo and radiation. The sores contributed to his inability to eat or swallow. The doctors prescribed what they called "magic mouthwash" for mouth sore relief. The solution is often comprised of these essential ingredients: an antihistamine to relieve pain, a local anesthetic to numb nerves and make them less sensitive to pain, an antacid to ensure all the ingredients coat the inside of the mouth, an antifungal, a corticosteroid to treat inflammation, and an antibiotic to kill bacteria. The mouthwash provided a small amount of relief, but it couldn't control the overall agony the sores caused him as they left marks like burns on his lips, his gums, his tongue, and the roof and floor of his mouth. Physically, three weeks into treatment, Jeff was noticeably different. His appetite had decreased at a rapid pace due to the nausea and mouth sores. He refused to eat most of the time, and his body began to shrink rapidly. Following lengthy arguments over his need for nourishment to avoid hospitalization, Jeff occasionally took a few sips of a smoothie or a nutrition drink to appease me.

Most days, intense nausea brought him to his knees for hours on our bathroom floor, where he lay on the cool tiles, often dry heaving and shivering as his body had nothing left to release. The weigh-ins at each appointment showed he was losing weight at an alarming rate. With Jeff not eating, we needed to find a way for him to consume nutrients, so we added weekly nutritionist appointments to our already daunting schedule. We had spent the few weeks between the surgery to remove the tumor and the start of radiation and chemo treatments attempting to increase Jeff's weight as much as possible, hoping to create an extra cushion for what was to come. Unfortunately, it only made a small dent. Jeff's lean frame would lose 25 percent of his starting weight that summer.

Trying to force him to eat and drink became a battle of wills between us. Those would be the first of many heated arguments between us during those years. His body and spirit were shattered as he was voluntarily torn apart every single day while we worked our way tremulously through that treacherous summer.

The summer wore painfully on, and the doctors became increasingly concerned that our strategy may have been too much for any person's body to handle at once. However, Jeff was insistent he would not stop until he'd finished every treatment. Supporting him tore at my heart and created a profound internal conflict. I wanted him to finish the treatments more than anything, but with weeks still to go, it seemed unimaginable that Jeff would be able to sustain the pace he'd been keeping without significant adverse effects.

Further consultations with the doctors and our nutritionist determined Jeff would need a feeding tube to continue treatments. The feeding tube would allow us to manually give his body the nutrition it needed by pouring liquid food into the flexible tube. There were many agitated discussions with our nutritionist, which ultimately made it clear that Jeff had to make a choice: either stop the treatments altogether or have a tube feed surgically placed in his abdomen.

In all his stubbornness, Jeff argued that he would figure out a way to drink the nutrition drinks. He did not want to walk with a pole attached to him or a scar on his upper abdomen where they would insert the tube. His pride was getting in the way. I knew he somehow felt that he had failed because he could no longer eat any nutrients on his own, but that was the furthest thing from the truth. He needed a gentle nudge of encouragement, reminding him how far he had come and that he was extremely close to the finish line.

Firmly but lovingly, I reminded him, "Honey, if you want to complete our mapped-out plan, you must have a tube inserted. You're not able to do this part on your own any longer. It's okay; you're not a failure."

We'd spent countless hours trying to find new food items that appealed to him and that he could swallow. He had been unbelievably strong and brave through it all, but still, he felt like he had let me down. I reminded him that to be strong enough to complete the treatments, the ultimate goal, he needed nutrients in his body to sustain him. I convinced him that he needed to accede to a feeding tube so he could focus what little energy he had on treatments and recovery, not on eating. Reluctantly, through tears of exhaustion, he agreed.

We made an appointment for the feeding tube surgery in the afternoon following his morning treatments. For the remaining weeks, Jeff now had an added challenge to carry with him each day. His strength and will to fight were unparalleled, but my heart hurt deeply with everything he courageously faced. The pole and bag of nutrients followed Jeff everywhere for the remainder of his treatments. During that time, I sensed his unwarranted humiliation as he pushed the pole along. Although I continually reminded him I was proud of his courage to fight, I could see in his eyes the stoic pride he once carried had been abandoned by the pole.

The man I called out at the pool in Las Vegas, his shoulders sturdy and muscular, deflated before my eyes. Day by day, his solid biceps and toned chest were reduced to flesh, merely clinging to bones. By the end of summer, his treatments were finished, and Jeff was unrecognizable. My sturdy, six-foot Canadian, who proudly walked into rooms exuding confidence, had been transformed in a matter of months. He had morphed into an emaciated and fragile figure that moved at a slow shuffle as he pulled the pole containing the nutrients his body needed to stay alive.

Through it all, our love was undeniable and unshakable. Looking into his eyes and feeling his touch was all I needed to remind myself of the man I fell in love with. One touch, and we found ourselves back in that pool in Vegas where our love bloomed. We held steadfast to our faith as our hearts regularly found the other through the torturous pain, breathing life into each other.

Our last day of treatment was July 27, 2018. Although it was our last day at Loma Linda, it was only the beginning and a small glimpse into our future. While his final chemo round was being administered, I slid back the baseball cap, now a part of his daily attire covering up the freshly balding scalp, and kissed his forehead gently. I read from our daily prayer book as we sat in silence and held hands, praying the chemo destroyed all the cancer cells.

When his chemo treatment was finished, we walked over to the radiation department for the final placement of his mask. Kissing his dry, brittle, and blistered lips before they securely fastened his armor one last time, I reminded him, "Honey, this is our last one; you made it. You're almost done. I'm so unbelievably proud of you. I'll see you on your last walk out to me." I could feel an enormous weight of relief slowly seep in as the tension in my shoulders softened, feeling the warmth of elation, knowing our nightmare summer was almost over. For the first time in months, I felt a sincere smile of joy find its way to my heart again. It was time to celebrate our victory for the summer of treatments we'd survived.

With a couple of hours of waiting time, I found a Party City store nearby to bring back a few balloons to celebrate his enormous accomplishment. I found ridiculously oversized heart and champagne bottle balloons. Initially, I thought it was a bit much since Jeff didn't like a lot of attention, but I realized that too much was perfect for the occasion. Oversized and over-the-top were definitely in order that day. As I took the balloons back to the car, hoping the heat didn't pop them, I was excited to drive back to the hospital knowing it was our last trip.

On my drive back, my phone rang with an unknown number. "Hello?" I asked. "Is this Stephanie?" an unfamiliar voice asked. "Yes, who is this? How can I help you?" The voice on the other end said they were calling from the insurance company. All summer, alongside everything else we were dealing with, I made weekly calls and updates with the insurance company to argue our case. The voice softened as she asked, "Is now a good time?" Annoyed to have that call interrupt our day of celebration, I let her go on, knowing that nothing would take away the happiness I felt that day. "Sure, today is a great day," I said. "Stephanie, we want to apologize for the past eight weeks. We have gone over everything, and I wanted to call you to let you know that the insurance will cover all of Jeff's expenses at Loma Linda," she explained.

I was blindsided and overwhelmed. The line was silent for a few moments while I composed myself, and then I blurted out, "Are you kidding me? Really? Are you serious?" For weeks, I'd made daily phone calls, sent emails, and held heated discussions, and I had finally given up all hope. I contemplated all our other options, including selling our home to cover the expenses. At that moment, I was speechless and utterly overcome with emotions that made me loudly burst into tears with her on the phone. I thanked her profusely for her efforts to make what we considered the best and correct decision. She apologized again for everything the insurance company had put us through that summer.

Back at Loma Linda, I was more ecstatic than when I'd left. Inside the hospital, I sat in my favorite waiting room chair. That particular chair brought me comfort during those hundreds of hours of waiting. The soft, beige leather was perfectly worn and nestled in a quiet corner; it offered the privacy I needed to journal and play peaceful music while keeping a watchful eye out for my love. I'd chosen that chair for the previous thirty-nine visits because it gave me a bird's-eye view of witnessing bravery walk toward me. I wanted to ensure that each time Jeff stepped out of that vortex of radiation, he knew there was loving support ready to lift him up, take him home, and cheer him on for the next day of battle. On that final day of treatment, as I watched his weak and broken body pushing the pole wearily shuffling toward me, his heroism was undeniable.

My emotions were bursting out of my chest. For the first time that summer, I could see a subtle lightness in him. With each step toward me, I could feel my heart swelling with hope and optimism for our future. I handed Jeff the large bouquet of congratulatory balloons. Wrapping into each other, we held on tightly, and then I tied the balloons gently to the feed tube pole so that everyone who passed us would acknowledge his irrefutable courage. That day, we would begin the healing of Jeff's body and our souls as we patiently waited several weeks to see if the risk we took, with the intense radiation and chemo schedule, paid off. We had done the work. It was time to recover and pray that everything we put his body through for eight weeks had been worth the anguish and suffering. Had it been the right choice and enough to accomplish our goal? Only time would tell.

Once the glow of hope settled in, I looked at Jeff. "Honey, I got a call from the insurance company today." Immediately, I saw his look of relief turn to annoyance; that was enough to take the wind out of his sails. I quickly interjected with the good news.

"Wait, Honey, it was a positive call this time. They are going to pay us back for all your treatments." Stretched to his limits, Jeff closed his eyes, bent his head down, and began to shake his head softly in disbelief as the tears slowly rolled down his sunken cheeks.

I knew the monetary gamble we took by putting the medical bills on credit cards had been weighing on him, too. We didn't often discuss the financial stresses. Instead, we saved our energy to get Jeff through the treatments. We focused on controlling what we could control. I reminded him it would all work out somehow; God always has a plan.

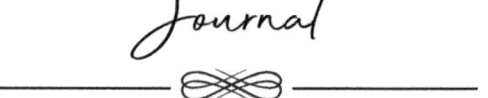

Sometimes survival means enduring a season that feels endless, trusting there's light on the other side. Write about a time when you or someone you love faced extreme physical, emotional, or spiritual hardship. What kept you, or them, moving forward, even when quitting felt like the easier option?

Chapter 11
RECOVERY

Making it through that first summer of treatments in 2018 was a living hell. It challenged and changed us in profound ways. Our love and bond solidified as we discovered a deeper appreciation and respect for each other, witnessing the remarkable resilience we each displayed. We shared our darkest fears and greatest hopes through vulnerable communication, connecting our souls to heightened depths. Our individual and joint efforts empowered us to continually fight to save Jeff's life and our love story. In the fall, while Jeff was still recovering, we marked off our first bucket list item. As luck would have it, the road to Big Sur had just reopened following a landslide. After Thanksgiving dinner with the family, we hopped in the truck and drove up Pacific Coast Highway (PCH), following the iconic California coastline. I drove, so between medications and resting, Jeff could soak in the breathtaking views of the looming cliffs to our right and the endless ocean to our left. With every turn on the winding road, our favorite tunes were cranked loud, the windows were down, and we breathed in the salt-kissed air and absorbed the sound of seagulls. The sun bounced off the truck's hood while an endless array of blues glistened in the ocean. We had no plan and no hotel reservations, only a destination and each other.

Pebble Beach, along the breathtaking "17-Mile Drive," was a visually stunning stretch of roadway that hugged the rugged coastline. As I glanced over at Jeff, I saw tears silently streaming down his gaunt face. He knew he wasn't physically able to play the course he loved so deeply, but he still wanted to be there—to breathe in the scent of freshly cut grass fused with the salty ocean air as we made our way toward the cypress tree guarding the eighteenth green.

The crisp fall breeze drifted through the truck's open windows, carrying the faint mist of the ocean roaring just beyond the fairway. Sea spray hung like a delicate veil suspended above the vibrant greens stretched endlessly before us. The amber sun hovered low in the sky, glistening on the perfectly manicured course. Jagged cliffs framed the edge of the water, their curves tracing the outer limits of where skilled golfers dared to play. But for us, it was about more than golf; it was about sharing a treasured moment.

We made our way to the distinguished clubhouse, wrapped in blankets and nestled into each other, shielding ourselves from the sharp ocean winds that whipped up with the setting sun. Sitting in the warmth of the fire pits with a glass of wine, we let the moment wrap around us like the blankets on our shoulders.

As the sun dipped toward the Pacific at The Links at Spanish Bay, a figure appeared in silhouette—his Scottish kilt swaying in the breeze and knee-high socks in full adornment. Then, the sound of the lone bagpiper began to rise, a haunting and mournful melody swelling across the fairway. The notes cut through the salt-tinged air, carried by the wind across the dunes and through the cypress trees. It wasn't just music but something more—a moment that left you suspended in quiet reflection. Guests paused in their steps as conversations faded. And for a few moments, everyone shared in the same stillness.

Captivated by every note, the bagpiper walked in rhythm across the fairways. Wrapped together, we watched the Pacific shimmering in the golden wash of the California sunset, and our minds drifted far away from cancer.

As a child, I often heard my dad, an avid golfer, speak with awe about the beauty of this course. To me, it became a legend—a far-off place that marked the pinnacle of the game. And now, sitting there in that sacred stillness, I, too, was filled with wonder.

On our way home, heading south along PCH, we felt like we stepped into a postcard as we crossed the iconic Bixby Creek Bridge. Its graceful arches connect the central coast to the north side, stretching across the canyon below, suspended between cliffs and sky. It was awe-inspiring.

The bridge, one of the most photographed landmarks on PCH, offers sweeping views of the rugged coastline, where jagged cliffs meet the restless sea and waves crash endlessly against the rocks below. It was the kind of view that made you pause, reminding you just how small you are in the face of something so grand and how full your heart can feel in a single moment.

We wound through the breathtaking curves of Big Sur and parked high above the ocean, the vast Pacific stretching out to our right. We stepped out of the truck. I stood in front of Jeff, nestling my back into his chest, his arms wrapped tightly around me. We closed our eyes and exhaled out all the exhaustion and despair. Standing there, we noticed a small road winding down toward the beach. We looked at each other without saying a word and decided to take one last detour.

With Jeff no longer needing a feeding tube for nutrition, the small, everyday simplicities in life found their way back to us. We grocery-shopped together again, and he could order from restaurant menus once more. We enjoyed the simple pleasures together as they began to stack upon each other. Our spirits started to heal, and we could feel the essence of our old lives slowly being restored.

I carefully navigated the truck down a narrow path toward the beach. We pulled out our beach chairs, a bottle of wine, cheese, and crackers for an impromptu picnic under the soft glow of the setting sun. The ocean breeze synced with the sound of the waves crashing against the rocky shore as our hearts soaked in the quiet joy of the moment and began to mend. The natural beauty of Big Sur and Pebble Beach renewed our souls while we slowed down and breathed in life.

Upon returning home from that rejuvenating first check on our bucket list, our hearts began to feel heavy, knowing that it was time for Jeff's first scans since that summer of hell. Praying for the best possible news but also bracing ourselves for the worst, we mentally prepared for Jeff's first MRI since the treatments ended. We'd tortured his body all summer, hoping for our best shot at buying more time, and had finally reached the moment of truth, the moment of learning if it had all been worth it.

It was time for the first MRI to reveal what remained of the monster we were battling. The results were both promising and terrifying. The tumors had shrunk in the areas we attacked and focused on all summer. This was encouraging, and it was a relief to know that the risks and the hell we'd put Jeff's body through were not in vain. However, our fears were confirmed: It was spreading rapidly. The scans uncovered that the cancer had metastasized to his brain, revealing new tumors that we needed to create a new plan to attack. These secondary tumors were similar to the primary tumor but in a different location. As time progressed, we discovered that cancerous tumors would relentlessly spread to Jeff's brain and spine. Our new normal was beginning.

Anguish settled in as we realized we would be reliving the same agonizing pattern from that hellish summer—again and again— in a desperate attempt to keep the unwelcome traveler at bay. Our lives would never be the same. Over time, it became evident that the cancer was spreading at a pace we would never be able to keep up with because doctors couldn't detect in advance where it was metastasizing. It reminded me of the game we played as kids, "whack-a-mole." We had to wait for the tumors to rear their heads so we could cherry-pick and tackle each one. It was rare that one tumor was detected at a time. Often, there were a handful of tumors that we needed to attack at once. Every two to three months, we trained ourselves. We learned to live with the inevitable diagnosis: Jeff was dying. We held onto hope in the corners of our minds, but deep inside, we knew the reality. It never got easier, but we created coping tools and training wheels custom- designed for each new diagnosis. We pedaled forward at a steady pace, never allowing each other to get stuck in those dark, muddy places for too long.

With each new full-body MRI scan every two to three months came days filled with anxiety because, for us, scans always brought more devastating news. It was never really a question of whether Jeff would be cancer-free or cured, although deep down, we always prayed to God for a miracle or a new treatment to be found. We didn't have the luxury to allow ourselves to believe the scans would come back clear. It wasn't pessimism but rather living in reality; it had been a terminal diagnosis from the start, and we could not ignore the probable, painful, inevitable ending.

We knew that forcing ourselves to live authentically was the only way to fight that enemy; we couldn't pretend it didn't exist or would disappear one day. We just needed to know how bad the most recent scan was, how far it had spread, and whether it was treatable. There was no cure, only hope for more time together and prayers for a miracle. Our new reality was to discover tactics to buy more time every few months.

Moving forward, our lives were filled with dozens of scans, custom-designed masks, and hundreds of radiation and chemo treatments that tore away at Jeff's fragile body just as he was beginning to find strength and recover from the previous treatments. Certain parts of our home resembled a triage center with machines, medications, and endless stacks of medical supplies needed to care for Jeff properly. It's funny how we have no idea of what we're capable of until we don't give ourselves a choice. When we look back at the whole, that's when the magnitude of the triumphs and all the layers hits us.

We didn't expect some of the unlikely collateral damage caused by the treatment's side effects. The many tumors and treatments wreaked havoc on Jeff's body. His eyes were the first victim. We continually bought new reader glasses to assist with his declining vision. Eventually, our ophthalmologist told us Jeff needed cataract surgery in both eyes. Then came shingles, which relentlessly attacked his back. We learned later that cancer patients are at a higher risk of shingles. Soon, he was struggling to hear, and we discovered that the aggressive treatments he'd been undergoing were destroying his hearing. We could substitute solutions for his hearing and vision, but we couldn't find a replacement for Jeff, so we continued with the treatments and dealt with the fallout as best we could.

With a new set of hearing aids and improved vision from cataract surgery, Jeff could continue to capture life experiences that brought him joy. It became a constant weighing of how far we could push the limits to keep him alive while maintaining a reasonable quality of life. We invariably balanced the cost of its extreme effects on his body with the perceived benefits. Even with the toll it was taking, we continued the aggressive cancer treatments. We both agreed the benefits far outweighed the cost, so we stayed the course.

We chose to look at life through a lens of hope and joy. This meant we kept our eyes open and found silver linings along the path during the years that the cancer challenged us. These moments brought light to our hearts and lifted our spirits, renewing our purpose of why we fought unwaveringly. It was spring 2019, and Jeff felt well enough between scans to join me while I took Jake on an East Coast college tour. The college tour coincidentally aligned with the Cancer Relay for Life rally, at which Maddie was asked to speak. While in college, she honored Jeff, her stepdad, by raising money to assist in cancer research. Maddie knew that it was unlikely that we could attend the rally. We were limiting added exertion for Jeff on an already tight schedule in the Northeast, and she was further south in Philadelphia. Knowing the weight and importance of the rally and how dedicated Maddie was to raising money for such a worthy cause, we rearranged our plans, made a fifteen-hour detour from our schedule, and took a train south to surprise her just as she was about to go on stage.

Tears of love and joy filled the room as Jeff and I found Maddie backstage. We were thrilled to sit in the front row with Jake, attentively listening to her heartfelt words describing her journey of witnessing the man she called dad battle a terminal diagnosis. Giving her speech at the rally, she surprised Jeff by bringing him up on stage and honoring him as one of Relay for Life's cancer heroes. Jeff never liked the spotlight, but that day, he shone like the hero he became.

The six months following the rally were filled with scans, treatments, and sprinkling in time to create special memories with loved ones. To us, those six months were neither cancer-free nor pain- and treatment-free, but they were some of the best months during those agonizing years. We found small pockets of freedom in between the treatments to enjoy life despite the cancer. We celebrated Jake's high school graduation and Jeff's son's college graduation, and we flew to Canada to celebrate Jeff's mom's eightieth birthday. We exceeded the original diagnosis and earned the joy of celebrating many milestones that only a year prior seemed unimaginable. Finding those beautiful moments through the pain renewed our spirits to fight for more time for Jeff to share with loved ones.

The summer of 2019 was coming to an end, and we had hit a good stride. Jeff felt more alive than he had in months. That didn't mean the cancer was in remission or that he was feeling like the man we all prayed he'd get back to one day, but it was something. It was just enough of a peak to give us a small window to live the life we loved, making memories at every opportunity.

The loop of scans and treatments never ended, but Jeff's body seemed to respond positively at times. In those pockets of hope, we made a few plans and stole little pieces of normalcy wherever we could, holding tight to the simple joys that reminded us we were still living, not just surviving. For the first time in over a year, we finally got a glimpse of our former selves and were excited to pack our suitcases for travel. We absolutely loved traveling together and everything that travel entailed, from looking on the internet for flights, hotels, excursions, cafes, and restaurants to embarking on the adventure itself. We both found so much pleasure in every detail. To us, both planning and traveling meant spending time together. Since the beginning of our relationship, time together had been one of our most prized possessions.

Never knowing if it would be our last adventure, we took advantage and soaked in every minute as if each trip was our last.

Following the cancer diagnosis, making plans meant booking flights and hotels days before departure. We had to wait until the last minute and assess if Jeff was feeling up for travel or even going to dinner down the street. Everything in our lives had become flexible and last-minute to accommodate this unwelcome traveler.

With Jeff feeling better, we got right to planning a trip. It was September, which meant one of our favorite seasons was upon us: football. Being Canadian, hockey was Jeff's first love, but football wasn't far behind. We decided to check off another bucket list trip and flew to Seattle for a quick weekend getaway with friends. That weekend, we soaked in all that Seattle had to offer.

On game day, we enjoyed the long walk over to CenturyLink Stadium. We arrived extra early and partook in every pregame festivity we could. Watching the teams warm up while drinking a few beers, we chanted and screamed along with all the other fans. Hearing the distant pulse of live music drifting through the air, we followed the sound toward the front of the stadium. It wasn't long before the rain began to sprinkle gently. Feeling the light mist, we stood with our ice-cold beers, listening to the live country band playing. Jeff tapped his toes with every beat of the music, a beer in one hand, the other hand stretched out high into the air as his fingers pumped to the beat. In a moment of rapturous glee, he turned and caught me smiling at him. Smiling back, he set our beers on a table and grabbed my hand. We two-stepped to a few songs as he spun me around, adding a few dips. During the final song, he dipped me deeply, then lifted me up and pulled me in for a long, slow kiss. We watched Jeff's favorite team, the Seahawks, and saw his favorite player, Russell Wilson, play a fantastic game. We loudly cheered on his team in the rain, wearing matching Seahawks jerseys. I will never forget watching Jeff in his jersey, his vibrant blue eyes taking it all in.

As we flew home from Seattle, we intertwined our fingers, our voices full of joy as we reminisced. The weekend had been filled with marvelous adventures, from Pike Place Market to the Seahawks game. Looking out the window at the majestic beauty of Mount Rainier below us, I felt our energy matched the elevation. There was a lightness I hadn't felt in months as we departed the plane in California. With the tension and stress evaporating, the overwhelming feelings of playfulness and spontaneity were afoot. It was as though no cancer existed, and the old familiar air of adventure seeped back in, enlivening our souls. Life felt easier somehow, the cancer less present.

We didn't want to lose the momentum from the invigorating experience we'd just had. We wanted to continue planning more hopes and dreams. Soaring from Seattle, we desperately wanted to continue the blissful joy of living and planning how we used to. We felt normal, at least as normal as one can feel when living with a terminal diagnosis as time is slipping away. Of course, there was no escaping the gentle reminders of cancer: the alarm clock for dozens of daily pills, the daily naps, and the slow pace we now took. I would carry some of these patterns forward following Jeff's passing, as I learned to appreciate life at a slower pace and add flexibility and spontaneity to it. During that period of our lives, we desperately longed for pockets of time, just like our time in Seattle, as they breathed life back into our depleted souls that cancer regularly drained.

Still on a high from Seattle, we threw caution to the wind and booked a trip to Boston. Jake had just started his first year at Boston College, and Parents Weekend 2019 was approaching. Maddie, being only a quick flight away in Philly, flew up and joined us. We spent a long weekend together at The Westin Hotel in Downtown Boston. It was another playful weekend as we filled our hearts with more unbelievable memories to hold. We explored the city's rich history and charming neighborhoods and ate delicious Italian meals that only the North End could dish up. We leisurely strolled through the narrow alleyways and uneven streets of Little Italy, where the smell of garlic and fresh dough wafted along the old-town streets. Endless market windows displayed rows of aged salami and fresh bread, while the cafes at every corner served up frothing cappuccinos as the machines steamed and hissed. While we waited in line at a restaurant, Jeff and Jake ran over to Mike's Pastry to pick up some of their famous cannoli. We all indulged in the sweet, flaky treats while we waited for our table. The contrasting beauty and aromas of the past and present filled our senses as we took in the authentic allure of Boston's North End.

We attended a Boston College football game on Saturday, our last night in Boston. Wearing our fan t-shirts, we tailgated with students and other parents who were there for Parents Weekend while we drank beer and danced in the parking lot. That night, we shared stories and laughed with the kids and strangers, who quickly became new friends. That day was Jeff's fifty-first birthday, and the game was a perfect way to celebrate. Following a fun afternoon, we hopped on the trolley and returned to the hotel.

Back at the hotel, we first stopped at the lounge for some water. Then, we wound our way through the maze of hallways and headed toward the elevator to our room. Jeff, with an old, familiar sparkle in his eye, suddenly reached out and tapped Maddie on her left shoulder as he zigged right, running past her laughing. Like children, the game of tag was on. Suddenly animated, I could see everyone getting revved up; Maddie and Jake yelled out and began chasing Jeff. Jake ran fast past them and into the elevator toward our room. Maddie was able to catch up with Jeff and tagged him as she raced down the hall toward the next elevator to escape the next tag.

It felt like years since I last saw Jeff display that kind of energy. He was hollering and bursting with laughter without a care in the world, running down the halls chasing the kids. At that moment, I forgot the fear and worry that cancer had brought into our lives; I saw my family playing, living, and embracing life, just like we used to. If Jeff was in pain at that moment, it was concealed by the sheer happiness coursing through his body; no one could have guessed he was between scans. The pure splendor was magnificent.

The two frolicking football weekends gave us an escape from cancer; they strengthened our foundations as we let down our guards to live in the moment. It was unreal watching Jeff run down the halls playing with the kids. Feeling the sheer freedom in Jeff's laughter, I watched them playfully run around chasing each other. My eyes filled with tears of joy as I witnessed the simplicity of the blissfulness we experienced that night. Life felt ordinary and positively familiar again. My heart soaked in every expression of their reckless abandon as I stood back at the end of the hallway while they raced forward, laughing and trying to catch each other. Observing the game of tag from behind brought so much pleasure to my heart.

I watched them turn a corner down the hall and couldn't see them anymore. Immediately, I felt tense, and a sense of foreboding came over me. I shouted out, "Be careful!"

Then I heard a thud.

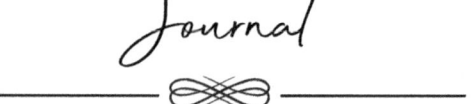

Recovery isn't just about healing the body, it's about finding moments that make your soul feel alive again, even in the shadow of uncertainty. Write about a time when you began to reclaim joy after hardship. What small, unexpected moments reminded you that life was still worth savoring?

Chapter 12

REARRANGE

Panicked by a thud on the floor of the hotel hallway, I thought, *Crap, who fell?* Speeding up, I took long, swift strides and quickly approached the end of the hallway.

In my motherly tone, I asked, "What did you guys do?"

I turned the corner and saw Jeff on the floor laughing and Maddie returning to help him up.

"Come on you guys, let's call it a night," I said. We all had early flights the next day, so it was a good time to wind down.

Maddie and I bent down to help Jeff up, but as we attempted to lift him off the floor, he screamed out in pain. We quickly realized he couldn't move. My mind raced with fear and thoughts of what could have happened to him.

"Honey, what's wrong? What hurts?" I asked.

He tried several times to get up, but with each attempt, he crumpled back to the floor with another excruciating cry of pain. Maddie and I tried to help him up from different angles, but Jeff still screamed out in pain. We were soon afraid to touch him again.

"Maddie, go get Jake," I demanded as panic seeped into my voice. We had escaped the burden of Jeff's illness during brief periods and occasional getaways. We compartmentalized our fears in order to live in the moment. But suddenly, we were forced to close the chapter on that playful weekend and abruptly return to our regular roles as advocate, caregiver, and patient. The joyful, carefree weekend swiftly dissipated in that hotel hallway. Cancer was center stage once more, reminding us how vulnerable and fragile life is as we tried to figure out how to help Jeff off the floor.

I realized we needed more manpower to lift him. Jeff was still gaining back some of the weight he had lost during treatments, but at six feet tall, he was more than Maddie and I could lift. Once Jake arrived, the three of us tried repeatedly to lift him, but it was useless. Jeff couldn't bear an ounce of weight without horrific pain. He was unable to bend his left leg, stand up on his own, or bear any amount of weight without screaming in agony. I wanted to call an ambulance, but Jeff insisted he was not going to the hospital. "We're on vacation, no doctors," he demanded.

Hesitant and trying to give him more time to feel free of hospitals, I agreed. I quickly came up with the idea of getting him onto the rolling chair from our room and wheeling him back to let him rest in bed. He refused to allow me to call for any help, so I apprehensively agreed that maybe with rest, the pain would pass. Jake ran and grabbed the chair, and we lifted Jeff onto it. He continued to cry out in pain as we wheeled him down the hallway, up the elevator, and into our room before finally lowering him into the bed. By the time we were all in our beds, the exhaustion from the last few hours felt crippling.

Too tired to change, we fell asleep, still wearing our stadium clothes. In the stillness of the dark room, I sensed Jeff wincing every time the bed moved. I tried my best to sleep entirely still, but it was no use; we both lay wide awake, pretending to sleep, trying to ignore what might be behind the pain. Finally, around 4:00 a.m., I said, "Honey, it's not a sprain or a small tear. Something is drastically wrong. I'm calling an ambulance."

In his monumental stubbornness, Jeff refused to allow me to call an ambulance. It took some convincing, but finally, I got him to take a cab to the closest facility, Tufts Medical Center. I called the front desk and asked hotel security to come to our room to assist us. We lifted Jeff onto the roller chair and wheeled him through the hotel and out the front entrance. Outside, we carefully moved Jeff into the backseat of a cab with his left leg sticking straight out of the window as he continued to groan from the pain. We made our way to the hospital with Jeff crying out at every touch of the brakes and acceleration of the car. I sat in the front seat with the concerned driver, my mind frantically speculating about what could have happened during the previous night's fall. It seemed incomprehensible to me that an ordinary event like a game of tag could flip our weekend upside down. All we wanted was to enjoy life without fear, like everyone else. As we left the hotel, I insisted the kids stay back and rest. They were exposed to so much with Jeff's diagnosis and the emotional anxiety that came with it, so I wanted to protect them as often as I could from witnessing the many unpleasant details of cancer.

Once Jeff and I arrived at the hospital, the emergency room staff began asking the usual questions. Our answers were more complicated than they had expected, as I listed every medication, treatment, surgery, and advanced healthcare paper. All the information locked into my memory led them down the path of our recognizable and turbulent road. It was painfully clear our vacation and short-lived freedom had come to a screeching halt.

When the scans came back, it was startling but oddly relieving. It wasn't cancer. Instead, Jeff had a fracture to his left hip and needed a hip replacement. A complete hip replacement might be devastating for most people, but for us, it was a relief. We'd become accustomed to life-and-death news and had prepared ourselves to hear the worst, but a hip replacement wasn't that. Still, it posed a considerable hurdle that Jeff didn't need to add to an overfilled plate, and we wanted to get the surgery over with quickly so he could start his recovery. We still had a six-hour flight between us and our home that proved impossible until Jeff's hip was fixed. Waiting for us at home was the next set of cancer scans; we had no time to waste.

We were shocked that the insignificant fall the night before had caused a hip fracture. Other than the cancer, Jeff was still relatively strong and healthy, so it made no sense that he could break his hip. The ER doctors were perplexed at first too.

Sitting in the hospital that day, I didn't want to deal with it all in an unfamiliar city, far from home. The thought of Jeff going through surgery and remaining in Boston for longer than planned as he recovered was too overwhelming to take in. But there was no other choice.

The doctors explained that what should have been a simple fall with bruising had turned into a complete hip replacement because Jeff's bones had likely been weakened during the countless treatments of radiation, chemo, and medication. We quickly settled into the reality that he needed immediate medical care; we'd become experts at adjusting to new realities. Far from home, a flood of paperwork, phone calls, planning, and worry set in once more, this time with a new team of doctors. What had started as an ordinary trip had turned into a devastating oddity, as cancer resurfaced to remind us that life for us was anything but normal.

Tufts took exceptional care of Jeff. They quickly scheduled him for hip surgery the next morning and then arranged his physical and occupational therapy for later that afternoon. After updating the kids and family in Canada and California, I realized I needed to return to the hotel, grab our bags, check out, and cancel our flights. There wasn't much anyone could do to help us. Jeff needed time to recover from surgery, and the kids needed to return to their lives. We were a year and a half into the cancer marathon, and I knew it would be full of unexpected miles that I couldn't handle alone. But this one, I could. As I gathered our belongings, I sobbed in the hotel room filled with birthday decorations and memories of normalcy. Packing up the room and reminders of our life back home was more disheartening than the hip surgery, therapy, and what lay ahead that week. The tears were not because we'd received unbearable news but because I didn't know if or when we might ever feel that exhilarating freedom of living again.

I took a round-trip taxi to the hotel and back to the hospital carrying all our luggage, feeling displaced and frightened. Once back, I piled up our bags in a corner of Jeff's room behind our privacy curtain. As the day wore on and the nurses became familiar, I shared a bit of our story with them, including Jeff's battle with cancer. Realizing I would need somewhere to stay while Jeff had surgery and recovered, I asked the nurses for hotel recommendations nearby so I could easily visit him. Typically, I would stay with Jeff overnight in the hospital, sleeping next to him on his bed or in a chair. But the room in Boston didn't have a chair, and I couldn't lie in bed next to Jeff with his painful fractured hip, so I had to find another option.

One of the nurses, who had taken to Jeff and me like we were family, quietly told us of a place at the hospital called the Cam Neely House, a beautifully furnished, transformed wing of the hospital. It's a respite for cancer patients and their families that a former hockey player, Cam Neely, founded in honor of his parents, who died from cancer. It contains sixteen studio apartments with kitchenettes, a group laundry room, and shared spaces for families being treated for cancer to watch movies and relax, all within the confines of the hospital.

We knew all too well what it was like for families undergoing treatment to drive every day, for months on end, to and from the hospital for treatments and the exhausting toll it took—scheduling, driving, waiting, and agonizing recovery, coupled with long drives week after week. The Neely House was a remarkable concept. The nurse shared that she wanted to call the Neely House to ask if I could stay there for the days following Jeff's surgery.

"The only way we will accept this generous offer is if a family going through treatments is not scheduled for one of the apartments, and the room would be empty this week," we told her.

Jeff was a cancer patient, but he wasn't going through treatments at that time. We were certain there was someone in far greater need than us who could benefit from the Neely House. Despite the blessing we knew it would have been for us to have a safe, convenient space to live while Jeff was recovering from surgery, we couldn't possibly take a room from a patient who needed it more than we did.

I stood beside Jeff, tightly holding his hand as the nurse's face filled with tears, "Do you know how rare that response is? You two need this; it's meant for situations like yours, too."

Our situation in Boston was stressful, but at that moment, we were well aware that others were battling far worse. Our battles would come—that was certain—but the hip replacement was a straightforward surgery that we needed to get through. The nurse called and found there were a few apartments open that week, so we gladly accepted the offer and were tremendously relieved.

With the apartment secured, I kissed Jeff gently on the forehead, grabbed our bags, and wheeled them through the hospital corridors. Never having to go outside the hospital, I could access a private elevator wing that opened to a place of peace and hope. Many signs of God's tender mercies were found throughout our cancer journey, and this was yet another.

Over the years, one thing I found incredibly useful for maintaining hope and peace was finding silver linings in every situation. It was like finding a needle in a haystack sometimes, but I knew I just needed to look around, and there was usually some positive that could be found in any circumstance that confronted us. Facing death daily was made slightly more bearable when we could unexpectedly slip away from the imprisonment of cancer to appreciate something beautiful or unexpected, even if just temporarily.

Maddie had returned to college in Philly, but Jake was just a short train ride away on campus and visited us daily. He kept our spirits up with laughter, fun stories, and a fresh set of eyes. One day, while he was visiting, I was hit with a beautiful silver lining: more time with my son. Jake's eighteenth birthday was that week, and I realized I could celebrate it with him in person. Jake and I cherish spending time together, so sharing his milestone birthday with him was perfect. We made dinner reservations at Legal Sea Foods in Downtown Boston. I sang him "Happy Birthday" over a mountain of ice cream with candles following a beautiful meal and a few lottery scratchers to commemorate his new adult status. Walking back into the hospital, I felt refreshed from spending invaluable time with my son.

Four days after having hip surgery, Jeff was discharged to stay with me in our apartment at the Neely House while finishing his physical and occupational therapies. Using a walker, we went through hospital corridors to our temporary home. I knew exactly what would bring a smile to Jeff's face once inside the Neely House, so I took him into the movie room. Hockey paraphernalia from Cam Neely surrounded rows of theater seating, and it was a delight for my Canadian. He reveled in looking at the signed jerseys, hockey sticks, and pictures while recovering. The Neely House offered me a peaceful space to strengthen my foundation and renew my spirits while Jeff recovered before flying home after that extra week in Boston.

With the doctor's approval, I rebooked our flights. I knew traveling across the country following an extensive surgery would be a considerable challenge, and the long, arduous flight home made me uneasy. Dr. Kavolus, Jeff's surgeon, contacted me to let me know he had called in a favor. He asked me to meet him and his colleague in a waiting room, where they handed me a box. When I opened it, they explained that it would help prevent further complications on our flight. Inside were chargeable air compression leg sleeves for Jeff to wear during the six-hour flight. Dr. Kavolus was concerned about blood clots during our long flight home, so soon after surgery. The compression sleeves would be our best bet to get him home safely. I embraced them both as I cried and thanked them for their gift and the kind, attentive care we had received throughout Jeff's stay.

Navigating the busy airport was complicated as we delicately maneuvered between volumes of people and luggage to ensure Jeff wasn't pushed or bumped. I wanted to wrap him in bubble wrap out of concern for the fragility of our situation. I gently helped him into a wheelchair so I could manage Jeff and our luggage simultaneously and carefully through the airport. Once settled on the plane, I put the compression sleeves on him for the duration of the flight.

We were relieved to finally be heading home following the successful surgery, and both had a much-needed, six-hour nap while in the air. But neither of us could hide our disappointment coming off two memorable weekends, only to end with an unexpected surgery. However, we would always remember with gratitude the kindness and care of those at Tufts and their profound impact on our lives, particularly in offering us a haven of reprieve at the Neely House throughout Jeff's ordeal.

Jeff's regular full-body MRI scans to detect the latest tumors were coming due upon our arrival home from Boston. Soon, our lives would be upended once more.

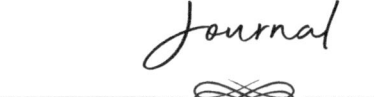

Sometimes life rearranges your plans in an instant, leaving you to navigate new realities you never saw coming. Take a moment to reflect on a time when everything shifted unexpectedly. How did you adapt, and what unexpected beauty or lesson revealed itself through the change?

Chapter 13
DELIRIOUS

Arriving home from Boston in fall 2019, after Jeff's hip replacement, we were faced with new tumors that were surreptitiously growing inside Jeff's body. From the time of our return, and throughout most of 2020, we found ourselves in a never-ending battle against cancer as new tumors were found and treatments were carried out. That year was filled with gloom and a constant sense of dread.

For nearly a year following his broken hip in Boston, Jeff spent the majority of his time at home, resting and recovering from treatments. When he did leave the house, it was often for the numerous scans, treatments, and endless hospital appointments. As the unwelcome traveler continued to take over Jeff's body, his days were lonely and his discomfort increased. He was home alone, living with an enemy that had profoundly rooted itself deep inside him, wrapped within every nerve and fiber of his body. I knew his days were quiet, and he felt separated from the world. He spent his time attempting to rest and manage the considerable pain he was in.

Each day, when I returned, I was excited to see him and spend evenings together, catching up and watching a movie. The distractions at work were welcome; they helped alleviate my isolation from the outside world most weeks. As the cancer advanced, our social lives dwindled. Jeff didn't have that option of a distraction, which made me feel miserable when I left each morning. When I returned home each day, I tried to lift his spirits by sharing stories about our business and details from my day.

One beautiful fall afternoon in 2020, I arrived home from work to find Jeff had set the stage for a quiet evening. A bottle of cabernet sauvignon rested on the kitchen island beside two glasses and soft-lit candles. It wasn't a special occasion—just one of the many loving ways he welcomed me home. These simple gestures carried me back to a time before cancer, when he always found thoughtful ways to ensure I felt his love. As I stepped inside, he met me with a look of quiet relief and warmth. His voice was tender as he said, "Hi Honeybee, I missed you. I'm so glad you're home."

He picked the songs and poured the wine, which helped fill our hearts with peace. I knew Jeff probably shouldn't mix wine with all the medications he was on, but I had learned over time which battles were worth clashing over. He insisted that he still wanted to enjoy the ordinary things in life and stated, "What's it going to do, kill me?" Although it was morbid, we laughed at the absurdity of that question.

The calming scent of lavender candles and the rich, fruity notes of the red wine were lost on Jeff. He hadn't been able to smell or taste since the summer of 2018, when intense radiation and chemo stripped those senses away. But it wasn't about smelling or tasting—it was about holding onto the simple joys he once loved, about finding ways to weave a sense of normalcy back into our lives. I couldn't deny him those small pleasures. In my eyes, he deserved anything that brought him even a moment of joy.

Before sitting with my wine, I checked Jeff's pill containers to ensure he'd taken everything that day. At the beginning of each week, I filled twenty-eight pill container slots with six to eight pills in each slot. We kept Jeff's medications hidden around the back corner of the kitchen. Though we could never entirely escape the imprisonment of cancer, we found small ways to mitigate the suffocating weight of it. Small subconscious acts like hiding his pills helped remove it from the forefront of our minds. We became skilled at leaving our thoughts of cancer on the counter next to the pills, tightly locked away.

After checking the pill containers, I was ready to enjoy the evening, knowing there were a few free hours before the next regimen of medications. I glided across the wood floors in my socks toward Jeff, picked up my glass of wine, and cuddled with him on the couch while we shared our days. Jeff told me how he went for a long walk around the neighborhood, took on some new hills, and did some tinkering in the garage, which he loved to do.

Shortly before sunset, something in Jeff's demeanor slowly shifted. He began to ask me the same question repeatedly, and I patiently gave him the same answer.

I asked him, "Honey, do you recall just asking me that?"

He replied, "No, I would remember asking."

At first, I thought the medications or the wine caused the confusion. But within minutes, it worsened exponentially, and alarm set in. Jeff's words became unrecognizable, sounds that didn't belong to any language I had ever heard. I tried speaking to him, but it was as if my voice didn't reach him. He seemed to be in a child-like trance, his eyes distant as he slowly pointed his index finger and traced circles in the air. Keeping my voice steady, I gently asked what he was trying to say. He looked at me and responded, but the words were nothing more than incoherent gibberish.

After a moment, he emerged from his state of confusion but had no recollection of what had transpired. He was sure I was exaggerating because he did not recall his words or behavior. I quietly grabbed my phone to videotape him to show the doctors what was happening. I wanted to be sure I wasn't overstating what was going on. I had hoped Jeff's confusion would pass, but it didn't, and I grew more concerned. While he continued going in and out of confusion and disorientation for fifteen minutes, I decided to call our doctors.

It was clear that something was very wrong.

I quickly had a doctor on the phone, described Jeff's behavior, and then gave him Jeff's vitals. With an urgency in his voice, the on-call doctor said, "Bring Jeff in immediately." Jeff insisted he was fine and refused to go to the hospital, but he had no choice. Every ounce of my being knew something was drastically wrong. This was one battle from which I would not back down. As stubborn as Jeff could be about certain things, I could be just as much of a force. He had learned to back down from me on certain battles over the years. I blew out the candles as we raced out the door, leaving half-drunk glasses of wine on the kitchen counter.

It had only been seven months since COVID-19 changed how the world lived. We vigilantly kept it away from Jeff, knowing his weakened immune system wouldn't survive that virus. With only patients allowed in the hospital, I knew I had a long night of waiting in the car ahead of me. We had adjusted to the strict COVID-19 hospital guidelines for the past seven months. That evening, I pulled up to the front entrance and got in the long line out the door filled with everyone wearing masks as I waited to check Jeff in. Once he had been checked in, I walked the grounds, went to the car, and tried to distract myself with work while waiting to hear from the doctors. My car had become my personal waiting room, sometimes for up to eight hours a day. It was long and grueling at times, especially during Southern California triple-digit summer months. Still, I knew it was nothing compared to what my love was going through inside the hospital.

The doctors immediately determined his condition was severe, although they didn't yet have a prognosis. They called to tell me I should go home. Jeff would be admitted until they could determine what was causing his symptoms. The doctors were highly concerned with what they were seeing. Hanging up the phone, I came to the frightening conclusion that there was more cancer in his brain. I thought to myself, as I had on so many other occasions, *Will this be the final bout with cancer that takes him from me?*

I had to control my curiosity and not google Jeff's symptoms, knowing the information available on the web would only make me more distressed. Over the years of battling cancer, I learned that most situations in life are temporary, and I can only control my reaction to the horrific circumstances we face.

It was times like that when I could feel my mind spiraling, and my circle of support kept me off the ledge. Being blessed with incredibly loving family and friends who were readily available was a saving grace throughout the journey. During moments of trial, I needed different types of support, so I created a "call list" in my phone notes that was easily accessible. I knew who "my people" were, but when panic sets in, we don't always think clearly, so having it written down was essential to me. My list included every person who gave me unconditional love—those who could lift me when I needed it most or simply let me cry. Someone to make me laugh, calm me down, or set me straight when panic took hold. When fear overwhelmed me, I didn't always need to talk; sometimes, just knowing someone was on the other end of the line was enough to bring comfort.

I have no recollection of who I called on that drive as my world once again threatened to crumble. There had been countless calls just like that one over the years we battled cancer. Unwittingly, my friends and family saved me from plunging into the abyss in my darkest moments. Releasing the exhaustion from my body, tears of worry made it challenging to see the road. Meanwhile, a calm voice on the other end of the line peacefully guided me home.

Arriving home, my breath heavy with exhaustion and my chest still tight from the drive, I gathered all the balled-up tissues in the car and sullenly walked inside. The weight of the night sat on my shoulders, pressing me further into silence. Scanning the house, I saw the remnants of what was supposed to be a calm and tender evening shattered around me. The air, still scented and wrapped in silence, was a haunting reminder of how our loving evening had spiraled into a nightmare of uncertainty and chaos. This was our life now—our new normal. At any moment, everything could change in an instant.

I sat bereft, surrounded by the dark loneliness of the kitchen, feeling exposed and vulnerable. Fighting back tears, I desperately searched for a glimmer of hope that might allow my emotions and mind to recover. Pouring a fresh glass of wine, I let my mind wander back to a memory of better times to ease my nerves. Opening my phone, I looked through our bucket list photo album. Stopping at one of our most memorable trips before COVID-19, I was reminded of our grand adventures during spring 2019.

We had traveled to Europe to celebrate the wedding of our dear friends Sean and Charlotte. A month before the wedding, Jeff felt well enough for the long international flight, so we excitedly began making plans. We could feel the energy building inside us as we mapped out the magnificent destinations for our next adventure. We never knew which check mark would be our last on that list, but we fought back the impulse to allow negative thoughts to seep in as we planned. We booked hotels and flights, choosing a highlight in each city—the Anne Frank House in Amsterdam and the Louvre in Paris—while letting the rest of the trip unfold magically each day. We found joy in slowing down, savoring each moment, and falling even deeper in love with each new experience.

At our doctor's appointment just before the planning began, our oncologist emphatically suggested we seize the opportunity while Jeff felt reasonably well. She didn't have to say what we knew: we were on borrowed time. The rare windows of opportunity would decrease as time progressed and could end at any moment. Initially, we were only planning to attend the Liverpool wedding. But with Jeff feeling reasonably well, we extended the trip to start in Amsterdam and Paris to celebrate our fifth anniversary, allowing ourselves time to cherish and soak in our first and last trip to Europe together.

With enough miles saved from our travels back and forth between Canada and the U.S., I upgraded our seats to ensure Jeff rested comfortably in his lie-flat bed. That choice allowed him to start the holiday without any unnecessary discomfort. We took in every luxury amenity from the first-class lounge, including enjoying a champagne toast to a phrase we had come to live by since cancer came into our lives, "Never let a diagnosis dictate your destiny." By that stage in Jeff's cancer, he was on the thinner side of the scale and was trying to put on more weight; Europe was the perfect place to indulge. We were so honored to be able to attend the wedding and watch the beloved couple take their vows as we all laughed and danced into the morning hours. It was a high point of our trip.

Closing the pictures and videos on my phone that fall night and bringing myself back into the present brought an unwelcome dose of reality that had been relentlessly depleting our spirits for months. Sullenly, I left behind the dark kitchen and walked upstairs to a quiet, lonely bedroom. I realized it was becoming a ritual as I lay down and tried to console myself to sleep. What had started as a soothing evening together disappeared before it got started. Temporarily avoiding reality and reliving those extraordinary moments in Europe had helped fight away my overwhelming worry and fear that night, but it was just a band-aid.

Journal

Life can turn in an instant, flipping moments of peace into waves of uncertainty. Think back to a time when your world was suddenly altered. How did you steady yourself, and what helped you find even the smallest anchor in the chaos?

Chapter 14
UNFORGETTABLE

A week passed, and we were still in the dark about what was causing Jeff's brain to spiral into a strange and unknown place. It was an incredibly lonely and desperate time for us both, with no solution and no physical contact. During that time, I often looked through old photos and sank back into those memories of better times as we traveled and shared our love.

Our travels through Europe before attending the wedding in Liverpool created two other memories that stood far above the rest. Rushing around to see everything was never our style of travel. We knew that wherever we traveled, we would never see it all. Instead, we chose to soak in moments and embrace the beauty of each experience at every turn. On our last day in Amsterdam, we returned to the hotel after exploring Haarlem, a quaint city in northern Holland, so Jeff could rest and refill his pills. Although Jeff's body during that trip was at one of the few peaks during those cancer years, he was always fighting the ever-present fatigue and pain. We kept with the tight medication schedule, never letting the pain get ahead of us, and allowed for plenty of time to rest in between all the walking.

Jeff had his nap, and then we were ready to leave the room to explore. Walking through the enchanting city one last time, we found our way to Vondelpark, a vibrant, urban park filled with acres of picturesque views of green landscapes, statues, and children's laughter. Amorous lovers nestled on blankets in the radiant, warm sun as summer beckoned. Billowy clouds painted the brilliant blue May skies. Mothers rode through the park in volumes with two to three children perched on the bicycle. The smell of cherry blossoms and tulips captured the essence of spring, evoking subtle freshness and a sense of blossoming beauty. It was a beautiful scene, engaging all our romantic senses.

We found a large, open spot on the grass next to a pond where Jeff had a few surprises he had tucked away. An endless romantic, he pulled out a blanket, a bottle of wine, paper cups he had grabbed from the hotel lobby, and a portable speaker out of his backpack. Jeff could turn an ordinary day in the park into the most memorable experience of my life. His gestures weren't usually grand, but they were always meaningful and showed me his heart—everything he did made me love and adore him.

A few hours away from the next pill alarm, we were thoroughly captivated by living in that moment. Jeff turned on the music and pulled up his custom playlist, "Jeffanie." We cuddled into each other on the blanket as we listened to some of our favorite country tunes, sipping from paper cups while stretched out on the grass in front of the pond. Jeff grabbed his phone, snapping pictures and videos as I poured wine, then I serenaded him. I sang one of our favorite Thomas Rhett songs, "Unforgettable." When the song ended, Keith Urban began to play "Making Memories of Us." Jeff stood up and put out his hand to help me up from the grass, and we slowly danced in the middle of the park.

That afternoon, we got lost in each other. Nothing could spoil the moment. Jeff's tender voice spoke to me while he videotaped, softly asking, "Whatchya doing, Honeybee?" My heart still skips a beat as the beautiful memories trickle down my cheek whenever I view that video. That day will be forever etched in my heart; it was truly unforgettable.

At the hospital, Jeff was still confused and hallucinating; his disorientation was noticeable to everyone but him. He became despondent and angry at his inability to understand the confusion we all saw. He was unable to recall the episodes of outrage and torment. When the two of us spoke on the phone or texted, he became increasingly irritated, not fully understanding why I couldn't come into the hospital (COVID-19 restrictions) to be with him. We both felt isolated, and he felt abandoned. Hopeless, but knowing there was little I could do to soothe his inability to comprehend, I was left to wait and pray.

Many days, I sat in the car for hours, working and waiting for those few moments when the nurse would wheel Jeff out to the large lobby window on the third floor so we could see each other while we talked on the phone. I brought framed pictures and balloons and made signs for the nurses to take back to his room to remind him he was not alone. I wanted Jeff to always feel the immense love and support he had on the outside. I could feel how much those minutes through the glass meant to Jeff. He was very isolated, and his spirits needed lifting to get him through the time in the hospital.

More testing was done to determine what was causing his confusion and disorientation. Finally, a spinal tap revealed that Jeff had viral encephalitis and swelling on two of the masses on his frontal lobes. Viral encephalitis is an inflammation of the brain. Additionally, he was diagnosed with brain necrosis, which reduced the blood flow to the brain. This can be caused by stereotactic radiosurgery (SRS). Jeff had received dozens of SRS radiation treatments to his brain and spine. Through the tests, it was detected that Jeff was having seizures, hallucinations, disorientation, difficulty speaking, and the inability to eat or drink. It was all caused by viral encephalitis and necrosis.

While we waited for medications to alleviate the swelling and mitigate his symptoms, Jeff begged me to find a way into the hospital. The doctors decided for his safety that they needed to monitor him with a hospital aide on watch twenty-four seven so that he wouldn't try to escape or hurt himself; he felt desperate and cut off as his confusion became increasingly persistent. With the seriousness of his condition, he was a risk to himself.

Watching him suffer, I wished for better days to come once more—days like the beautiful ones we'd spent together in France the year prior.

Leaving Holland, we took the speed train to Paris to stay at the Westin Vendôme, ideally situated in Paris's exciting first arrondissement. We sat with our delightful concierge, who wanted to discuss our trip as she got acquainted with us. We shared that it was our fifth anniversary celebration that week in Paris and how we had planned the trip at the last minute. We learned a bit about her life in Paris as well. By the end of the conversation, a palpable energy of romance took over. As her eyes lit up, she handed us our room keys with a broad smile stretching across her face. "I put you in a room that I'm sure you will love," she told us.

We exited the elevator and made our way to a private corridor leading to a set of grand doors, unlike any other doors we had walked by. We opened the oversized double doors with large, shiny brass knobs that took two hands to hold. Standing in the hallway, we looked at each other and started to smile, feeling something magical behind those doors. And there was.

We pushed our way into a large bedroom suite with a sitting area. Two sets of French doors draped with thick, elegant curtains stood in front of us across the room, placed on either side of a fireplace. We put our bags down and crossed the room to open the doors. We found ourselves looking out to the Louvre and the Jardin des Tuileries next to it, with the Eiffel Tower as our backdrop. Sitting on a small table next to the French doors were champagne and macarons waiting for us. It was the ideal fairytale setting for a romantic five days in Paris. That afternoon, we kept the French doors pulled wide open and breathed in the scent of cherry blossoms and the fresh smell of spring as we cuddled into each other, looking out to the Louvre and the Eiffel Tower. We later found our concierge and thanked her for the beautiful room upgrade; it was more spectacular than we could have imagined.

We spent the week strolling through the streets of Paris, soaking in the city's beauty and romance. We looked at priceless art and historical sites, sat in cafes each day, and completely immersed ourselves in the city of love. On our last day, our fifth anniversary, we hired a photographer named Alex to capture our experience in the captivating city. What was supposed to be a one-hour photoshoot with Alex turned into four hours of frolicking through Paris as we hopped into one Uber after another around the city. He captured romantic shots around the hotel and from our balcony as we held champagne glasses and looked out at the Louvre and the Eiffel Tower. Initially, we'd planned an early dinner following the one-hour photo shoot, but Alex had other ideas, so we delayed our dinner. During the conversation, Alex asked us about our lives, and we shared our love story and how special that trip was because we were on borrowed time. Anyone who met Jeff could see he was battling something; he politely asked us a few questions regarding Jeff's health, and our friendship with the photographer blossomed. Alex asked if we would like to take more pictures around the city, and we explained that we didn't budget for a half-day photoshoot. "This one is on me," Alex insisted. We happily accepted his kind offer and changed into something special for the occasion. We took off in an Ubér, placing complete trust in our new Parisian friend as he took over the remainder of our anniversary day. With our photographer riding along with us, it felt like the world-famous city was our playground. We could feel a magical afternoon had only just begun.

At the first stop, we entered a hidden neighborhood with Parisian architecture walls that lined a cobblestoned corridor. Alex had us walk around as he observed us in conversation. Next, we traveled to a bridge beside the Eiffel Tower. I wore the heels I had packed for the wedding and Jeff's favorite blue dress, which matched his eyes; he looked dapper in his soft pastel dress shirt and slacks. This was a version of ourselves that we had lost to cancer, but not in Paris. On that magical day, our talented photographer found the laughter in our eyes, the tenderness in our hearts, and the passionate devotion we held for each other while we strolled playfully through the streets next to the

Eiffel Tower. Mercifully, the only thing not captured in the hundreds of photos was our fear and exhaustion from cancer. It was remarkable how he encapsulated all the beauty and none of the beast that lay below the surface.

The golden sun dipped low over Paris, drenching the city in hues of amber. The Seine River shimmered like liquid gold as the sky melted into soft lavender, casting our shadows over the cobblestone streets where quiet laughter was shared between lovers. The Eiffel Tower stood tall in the distance as an intoxicating blend of velvety espresso, fragrant spring flowers, and wine swirled in the air around the city, rich with history. The world felt hushed, as if the city was holding its breath, pausing just for us.

Each picture made the city look and feel abandoned. We took an Uber to the Jardin des Tuileries and the Louvre grounds. Alex soon learned we loved to dance, and he wanted to capture it. We played music from Jeff's phone, and in the middle of the dirt and gravel grounds where Napoleon once rode horses, Jeff spun me around as my silky blue dress flowed and twisted with every turn.

The evening of enchantment continued as we walked over to the Louvre's glass pyramid. The sun was setting, and the ominous blue and gray sky lit up our surroundings, with the threat of thunder looming. Jeff and I walked through the grounds holding hands, talking, and stopping for a kiss occasionally while Alex captured it all in the City of Love. We strolled the grounds of the Louvre under the moonlight with barely another soul in sight, then wandered through the promenade into hidden hallways as Jeff held me tightly, walking over the cobblestones so I didn't trip in my heels. With the clouds threatening to bring on a storm against the moonlight, Alex honored our love. It was a perfect way to preserve our once-in-a-lifetime trip. The Paris photoshoot encapsulated us passionately in love, like a scene from our very own fairytale. Compartmentalizing our fear to embrace joy in the moment was essential to preserving our sanity during those years.

Alex celebrated our love story in ways we never imagined. Having those photos to reflect on allowed my mind to drift into beautiful memories, often bringing hope back into hopeless situations.

Now at the hospital battling a ruthless enemy, I felt helpless—light-years from the romance and magic of Paris. I desperately tried to gain admittance into the hospital every day since I'd dropped Jeff off. I respected the protocols but became increasingly concerned about Jeff's mental state. With every call and text, I feared that he could harm himself, not realizing what he was doing. My patience was wearing thin as I heard the desperation in his voice every day, asking where I was and not understanding why I couldn't be with him. He needed comfort and familiarity. Finally, after a week, our doctor was able to get me into the hospital with strict rules. I had to test negative for COVID-19, and once inside, I was not allowed to leave. I immediately gathered everything I needed for an extended stay and raced to City of Hope Hospital to be with Jeff, grateful to comfort and calm him.

We spent the next week together in the hospital as the swelling subsided. Jeff had been in for two weeks when we could finally return home together. We were relieved to be back home, but the impact of the damage and continuous swelling to his brain that we attempted to manage dramatically altered Jeff. The new drugs prescribed to treat the encephalitis would permanently be added to his already long list of medications.

Upon returning home, there was a noticeable turning point in Jeff's quality of life. The unexpected extended hospital stays became more frequent, and his ability to rebound and recover continually declined and became almost nonexistent. There would be no more checks on our bucket list. That nightmare we'd endured during Jeff's battle with encephalitis was merely one of many hospital stays that awaited us over the next ten months. This was all a direct result of Jeff's cancer and the damage from the treatments that relentlessly tortured his weakened body. We knew in the darkest parts of our hearts that Jeff was terminal. That was an integral part of our daily lives. However, we never anticipated the tragedy that lay ahead of us.

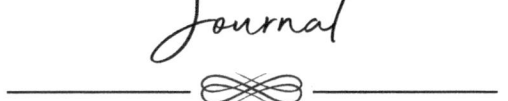

Some memories are so vivid they feel like they're stitched into the fabric of who we are, carrying us through even the hardest days. Think about a time when joy felt so pure it eclipsed your worries; how can you hold onto that feeling and let it fuel you during seasons of uncertainty?

Chapter 15
SPIRALING

On May 16, 2021, the night before our seventh anniversary, I could see that Jeff was feeling tenuous. Oftentimes, he put on a façade that I could see right through; it had become painfully noticeable that we could no longer control or hide the torture he was enduring. The disease was clearly gaining the upper hand. I didn't question him during those times, not wanting to take away the last remaining dignities where his valor and chivalry could shine through.

He unconvincingly attempted to be excited about making dinner plans for our anniversary the next day, lovingly saying, "Honeybee, I'll make a reservation so we can have a romantic dinner out tomorrow night; you deserve a special night out."

All I could think of was how he deserved a night where he could once again eat the foods he enjoyed, sit through a meal pain-free, and not feel the sharp agony that constantly destroyed all the ordinary comforts he used to enjoy in life. I wanted so badly for Jeff to partake in everyday activities without the side effects of cancer taking away the simple pleasures. My heart broke into hundreds of pieces because I couldn't take his suffering away; nothing could.

By that time, his entire body was relentlessly tormented. The cancer was merciless. Although the medications were adjusted and increased weekly with our pain management team at City of Hope, the cancerous tumors were aggressively attacking his brain and spine. We couldn't adjust the pain medications fast enough to give him any relief, as the monstrous cancer was always a few steps ahead of us, wreaking havoc on his already fragile body. With full-body MRI scans every two months, we'd detected dozens of new tumors in Jeff's brain and spine over that past year.

It was spreading rapidly. We fought each one as diligently and forcefully as if it were the first tumor. By that point, Jeff's body was saturated with hundreds of treatments: radiation, chemotherapy, and immunotherapy (a type of treatment that helps the immune system fight cancer). Jeff's medications consisted of high dosages of Norco, OxyContin, fentanyl patches, dexamethasone, and gabapentin (for the extreme nerve pain that coursed through his entire body, from his feet to the nerves in his teeth), to name a few. There was not an inch of Jeff's body that wasn't in excruciating pain every day.

Additionally, the high levels of so many medications altered Jeff's personality, which brought on extreme aggressiveness, irritability, memory loss, and erratic behavior. I reminded myself not to take it personally when he acted or spoke in ways that were out of character. If I felt provoked by the new version of Jeff, I relied on close friends and family to talk me off the ledge so I didn't take out my frustrations on him. He was dying, and he did not need or deserve to be admonished for something he couldn't control. I was losing the love of my life before my eyes each day for over three years, and my patience and tolerance levels were also fading with each passing day. I could feel myself becoming easily agitated at things I'd usually take in stride. I could see a new, temporary version of myself emerge. Expectedly, with both of us dealing with life and death each day, there were moments we went head-to-head, but we always returned to our center, our love for each other.

It had been months since Jeff had truly enjoyed anything. His overall condition went drastically downhill the previous fall when he contracted encephalitis; the damage had significantly impacted his quality of life. As time wore on, his condition progressively worsened, and the hospital stays for various ailments became more frequent, including one severe condition caused by a chemo cocktail that caused his lungs to collapse. Every two to three months, for a few days to a couple of weeks, he was admitted to the hospital for an unexpected condition.

While he was planning our anniversary dinner for the following evening, I sensed a new frailty and decline in his demeanor. I played along because I'd learned that whatever demon the cancer was threatening below would surface soon. So, instead of asking him if he felt well enough to go out, I amenably said, "A romantic dinner sounds lovely, honey."

I had hoped to wake up before Jeff the next morning, but as I rolled over in bed on Monday, I saw he was already awake. He often slept in much later than me; his body needed immeasurable amounts of rest. His exhaustion from the cancer was compounded by his inability to sleep through the pain. He was up almost every night, either pacing, trying to walk through the pain, or asking me to massage out the spasms in his back, arms, or legs. The agonizing aches and pains were getting more intense, and he was sleeping less and spending many hours alone in the moonlight, working through the pain. Most nights I felt helpless, and the only support I could offer was to comfort him in bed with warmth and prayers. Watching the once-vibrant man wander our home aimlessly like a lost child broke my heart. Over the past handful of months, the longevity and severity of the pain had increased exponentially.

This unwelcome traveler steadily found new places to infiltrate and torture Jeff, and we couldn't slow down the pace. The steroids he took to combat the swelling in his brain caused extreme weight changes. Jeff's average weight was 170 pounds. During our battle with cancer, he fluctuated between 130 and 215 pounds, which created added distress. All the medications and treatments transformed and warped his body, making him almost unrecognizable. His walking became a slow shuffle, and the newest menu of tolerable foods became increasingly limited. The quality of life Jeff once knew had essentially become nonexistent.

What more could be taken from him? I thought to myself.

Before I could lean in to give him a happy anniversary kiss that Monday morning, I could see he was struggling to breathe. I calmly asked him what was happening and how long it had lasted. He explained that he struggled to breathe most of the night. With Jeff's background as an ICU respiratory therapist, he was highly knowledgeable in that department, so I deferred to him, the doctor and patient rolled into one. We tried several ideas Jeff suggested, such as a humidifier and hot steam. Nothing offered any relief, and as time passed, his breathing became significantly more labored.

"Honey," I exclaimed hesitantly, "I need to call our doctors."

I knew he wanted the day to be romantic and memorable and would resist calling the doctors. We desperately wanted to enjoy that day and could feel the heaviness that it could very well be our last anniversary.

Jeff insisted it would pass, but there was a drastic change within minutes. My instincts couldn't listen to Jeff and ignore what I knew in my gut, so I called City of Hope. I tried not to panic, but he was gasping for air, and the shortness of breath made it difficult for him to speak. He could barely breathe. I could feel the fear setting in again, but I forced myself not to feel and instead to act. It was not passing on its own, and I was not equipped to handle its downward direction.

I described the symptoms to the nurse on the phone, and she asked me to test his oxygen level. I pulled out our pulse oximeter (an electronic device measuring the blood's oxygen level) and relayed that his oxygen level was below 70 percent, which was life-threateningly low. Though I had no medical background, I'd learned a lot over those years. Still, I was not trained to handle all the situations that we continually encountered, so I relied on our trustworthy team at City of Hope.

Despite the nurse's calm voice, I sensed alarm. She immediately instructed me to call 9-1-1 for an ambulance and then hung up. My heart began to pound, and panic set in once again. Heat rose through my body as my hands began to sweat, and my mind raced. Fight-or-flight mode kicked in, and I frantically told Jeff I was dialing the number. I had never needed to call it before.

Jeff stopped me as I started to dial, "Do—not—call—an—ambulance," he said, gasping for air.

I started arguing with him, but he was agitated and yelling at me not to call 9-1-1. With the terror of him not being able to breathe, there was no time to argue.

Overwhelmed with fear and frustration, I yelled, "Fine, get in the car now!"

We couldn't waste a single moment arguing; we had to move quickly. I gathered what I could, then slowly and carefully helped Jeff down the stairs. His body was weakening rapidly; whatever strength he still possessed was quickly vacating his body.

Barreling out of the garage, I raced down the freeway frantically, with fear-filled silence engulfing the car. The only thing that could calm the tidal wave of intense fear building inside me was to reach back into my bucket of beautiful memories; they were bittersweet in that moment because I felt it could be our most tragic anniversary. Those special memories brought me to a place of peace and joy, where I could drift away and vacantly recollect the wonderful life we once enjoyed together.

A memory of our first anniversary drifted into my mind. Jeff had planned a romantic getaway to the Jasper Park Fairmont in Canada. The rustic log cabin rooms were a dream, with wood-burning fireplaces for cozy nights cuddled into each other. Situated right next to the lake, our front door opened to the sight of majestic elk greeting us as we stepped outside.

We spent an afternoon canoeing on the magnificent lake cradled by the breathtaking Rocky Mountains. The crisp mountain breeze carried the aromatic scent of pine from the vast wilderness surrounding us. Abundant wildlife stirred along the water's edge, adding a quiet magic to the already romantic setting. As we glided through the stillness, the crystal-clear water revealed smooth stones and soft moss resting on the lakebed beneath us. The majestic Rockies towered around us, their snow-capped peaks mirrored perfectly on the glassy surface—a reflection so vivid it felt like we were floating through a painting.

May in Canada can be quite cool, but to us, it was perfect. The lake was ours alone as we paddled across its still surface, watching the ripples fan out in gentle rings around us. We glided from one side to the other, serenaded by the music from Jeff's playlist, which echoed softly over the water. The snowcapped mountains reflected in the lake created a breathtaking scene that felt fake. My photos appeared so surreal that my friends later accused me of photoshopping us into a dreamlike backdrop. But that was our life together, beautiful and unreal.

Jeff and I spent the entire day on the lake, soaking in the Canadian Rockies, their beauty encircling us for hours. We stopped in the middle of the lake, and I thought it was the perfect moment to toast the man I knew I would spend forever with. Carefully, I stood up in the canoe, steadying myself to avoid tumbling into the icy water, ready to make an anniversary toast. But just as I began to speak and tell him how much I cherished our life together, Jeff gently interrupted. Unbeknownst to me, he had already started videotaping. He spoke softly into the camera, his voice tender, his eyes never leaving mine.

"You're the most amazing woman I have ever met; I'm the luckiest person in this world. Honeybee, I honestly, truly love you, sweetheart." My heart melts all over again every time I listen to the tape from that day. In the video, I stood in the canoe surrounded by the glorious scenery of Jasper, Canada, as a smile widened across my face. I was beaming, radiant with love, as I listened to Jeff share how much he adored me and our life. We spent that weekend soaking in the awe-inspiring natural beauty, watching herds of deer, elk, and caribou graze along the roadside, and hiking the trails around the magnificent Athabasca Falls. My heart was floating. We soaked in every moment on that first anniversary, not realizing what our future held.

I pulled up to the emergency room entrance and was slammed back to reality. Our lives had become anything but romantic and beautiful. Instead, we faced Jeff's impending death every day. With the time between each hospital stay becoming more frequent, I sensed the shadow of death gaining the upper hand, closing in on us with each passing moment.

Frantically, I ran to the entrance and asked for help with a wheelchair; Jeff was too weak to walk on his own, and I wasn't able to support his weight. After getting Jeff situated at the hospital, still following COVID-19 protocols and unable to go in, I pulled my car into the closest lot, where I sobbed uncontrollably. When I finally composed myself, I felt on edge and needed to occupy my mind from the worry. I cautiously left the hospital grounds and went to fill up my gas tank. Any small task was a helpful distraction while I waited for a call from the doctors. Just as I finished pumping gas, I received a call from an unknown number.

I answered the phone, and a person on the other end abruptly interjected, "Is this Stephanie?"

Standing beside my car door, pumping gas, I asked, "Who is this?"

"Stephanie, I'm the surgeon with Jeff right now."

"Wait! What?" I interrupted as my panic soared. "A surgeon, for what? Jeff had an issue breathing; he didn't need surgery, he'll be fine. What's going on?"

"Stephanie, how far away are you?" he interrupted.

I was about fifteen minutes away. The surgeon, in an alarming voice, instructed me to return to the hospital immediately.

"We need to take Jeff into an emergency surgery, and he refuses to go in unless he gets to see you and talk to you first."

"I'm on my way," I quickly said.

"You need to hurry; he doesn't have much time; please drive safely," the surgeon cautioned as he hung up the phone.

I was hysterical as I drove back to the hospital. I don't recall anything; I was paralyzed, but somehow, I safely arrived.

I know I made a call as I drove. I needed someone to try to keep me calm, but I don't know who I called; I just knew I needed another voice regulating my hysterical state as I sobbed tears uncontrollably.

I thought to myself, *God, was this it? Would he still be alive when I arrived at the hospital? Not like this. I need to see him; I'm not ready. I need to hold Jeff one more time. We had dinner plans tonight to celebrate our anniversary. Would I be planning a funeral instead?*

I remember ripping into the parking lot and going to a side trauma entrance for drop-off only. Over the years, I had memorized every inch of the parking lots and hospital corridors. I threw my car into park and left my purse, keys, phone, and everything else in the car. Only one thing mattered: getting to Jeff.

A nurse was waiting for me. She grabbed my arm and swiftly guided me down a hall and into a private room to see Jeff. I had no idea what to expect. I saw him on a bed, being prepped for surgery with IVs and an oxygen mask. I felt grateful and crushed all at once. *Thank God he's still alive*, I thought. But something was drastically wrong. His demeanor was innocent—as soon as he saw me, he appeared childlike, and we both began to hold each other, crying desperately.

Feeling sick and alarmed, I asked, "Honey, what's going on?"

At this point, it was becoming increasingly difficult for him to speak; he could barely put two words together at a time. His eyes filled with tears, and he tightly grabbed my hand. I could feel all his strength.

He pulled off the oxygen mask and said intermittently, "Honey—bee—they—need—to—put—a—tracheotomy—in—me."

Having been a skilled ICU respiratory therapist for years, Jeff knew exactly what that meant. It was one of his worst nightmares. Cancer ripped away every inch of his dignity piece by piece. Jeff had said to me on more than one occasion during the many traumatic hospital stays, "I never want a trach put in me; I know what that life looks like in detail, and I will not have that done to me."

Jeff's demeanor shifted from an innocent child looking for guidance to a man filling with rage over what he was facing. Unable to form words, he looked at the doctors and nurses and sternly motioned for everyone to leave. When it was just us in the room, he looked at me with a distinct disappointment in his eyes, carrying the weight of words left unsaid of our brutal reality.

Knowing we were under the clock and that they wanted to take him in immediately, Jeff once again took off the oxygen mask to form a few words at a time in between the breaths.

With discouragement in his voice, he said, "Honey—bee—they—want to—put—a—trach—in—me," as he gasped for more air. Taking a few hollow breaths from the oxygen mask, he went on, "NO, I—won't—have—that—you—cannot—let them—put—a trach—in me."

Before I spoke, I tried to gather my thoughts through the sobbing. It was a defining moment, a crucial decision that needed to be made in a matter of seconds, and it was life and death.

My mind rapidly flipped through scenarios, and my thoughts went wild with questions:

Do I ask him to go forward with a procedure that terrified him and would require more bravery as it added to the long list of the countless collateral damage his body had already endured from cancer?

How could I ask him to take away more of his dignity and watch his mind and body be destroyed?

But if he didn't do the surgery, he would die. Was he ready to die? Was I ready?

Were we prepared to say our final goodbyes?

Knowing he was looking to me for guidance, I somehow gathered enough strength to pull myself together.

Through sobs, I gently but firmly asserted, "If you don't do this procedure, you will suffocate; it's that simple."

My weeping was irrepressible; I could barely speak through my fear. "If you don't want the trach, you don't have to, but if you don't do the surgery, then this is it. You will die today, Honey."

It was one of those out-of-body moments when I flipped a switch, sharply turned off my emotions, and became clinical.

I wiped away the tears and firmly stated, "What do you want to do, Honey?"

My heart sank with each syllable.

What quality of life would remain? I thought. For Jeff to live with a tracheotomy seemed intolerable. Balancing my caregiver, lover, and advocate roles required finesse and patience. I knew what we both wanted, always and forever more time, but that was rapidly slipping through our fingers. Wearing incongruent hats was often a delicate juggling act. The balance of being practical and clinical to accomplish tasks decisively, frequently, and harshly contrasted with what our hearts wanted. It had become an endless test of my strength to balance those roles and come out feeling confident in our decisions. I learned to quickly weigh all the options within seconds and reach a thoughtful and rational resolution. Guilt or second-guessing had no place in our lives by then. Immediate and decisive decisions were required.

I could see in his eyes that as much as he did not want the trach, he was not ready to say his final "I love you." He looked at me desperately with tears in his eyes, dropped his chin to his chest, and shook his head from side to side in disbelief. He was broken. He needed me to make the call, so I did.

In five days, we would've been in Nashville, taking Jake on a campus tour before he transferred to Vanderbilt University and then flying to Philly for Maddie's college graduation. Knowing Jeff was declining quickly, we had planned and booked the trip hesitantly. He had been so excited to attend those momentous milestones. That was the last time we planned a trip.

The flights were booked to celebrate those significant achievements. We were so proud of both Maddie and Jake. The year following Jeff's diagnosis, we were able to attend both of our sons' college and high school graduations; each milestone we were able to experience together was a gift. He didn't want to miss a single one of them. We'd been so excited about the trip to Nashville that we had bought advance tickets to see the Grand Ole Opry, another item on Jeff's bucket list. That day in the hospital, we begrudgingly agreed to have the tracheotomy surgery, knowing it meant there would be no more milestones Jeff could attend. We were fully aware that our bucket list would not see another checkmark.

I called everyone in Canada with yet again more devastating news. His mom and sisters were always incredible at stepping up and helping us when things got rough, flying down to provide extraordinary support. That was another one of those times. It was so difficult for his family to live two thousand miles away, knowing how severe Jeff's condition was, but there was nothing we could do to change the distance.

The surgery was successful, but the doctors wanted to keep him in the hospital to monitor him for the week. We were due to leave for the East Coast in just a few days. Once Jeff's family arrived, they insisted that I fly with Jake to tour the college, enjoy Nashville, and continue as planned to attend Maddie's graduation in Philly. In my mind and heart, there was no way I could leave Jeff in a hospital in that condition and fly across the country, let alone enjoy time away while he lay in a hospital bed for a week. In the end, the doctors, Jeff's family, and mine all but forced me to get on that flight. Jeff convinced me he would be fine and that I couldn't miss those milestones.

I was extremely conflicted, but because there were plenty of direct flights to LAX, I knew I could return in just a few hours if necessary. When I said my goodbyes to him at the hospital, we held each other tight as I leaned in to hold and kiss him; the tears poured out of me, knowing there was a slight chance that I may never see him again. I carried a deep and heavy guilt over leaving him there. He slowly covered the trach hole with tears in his eyes and reminded me to enjoy myself and hug our girl at her graduation. Jeff's selflessness was remarkable.

Walking through the airport, I was weighed down with guilt, wondering if I would see Jeff again. A tightness was building in my chest along with a familiar lump in my throat. I held back the tears just long enough to find my seat. Jake could see I needed space as I longingly stared out the window and quietly played mine and Jeff's favorite songs on my headphones. I closed my eyes, allowing myself time alone with my thoughts. As we took off from Orange County airport over the ocean, tears poured out of me uncontrollably. I sat in my seat that morning, praying the sound of the jets would mask my weeping, and I begged for mercy, hoping that it had not been our last kiss goodbye.

Journal

Sometimes we are called to make impossible choices, ones that feel like they carve pieces out of our hearts. Take a moment to write about a time when you had to act quickly under pressure, even while your heart was breaking. How did you find the strength to move forward, and what did you learn about yourself in the process?

Chapter 16
STRETCHED THIN

I increasingly turned down social invitations due to Jeff's declining health following his cancer diagnosis in April 2018. But on Father's Day weekend 2021, my parents were having a family barbecue, and I wanted to attend to spend time with my dad. I knew Jeff would not be able to join me, so I planned to go during his afternoon nap.

During the first couple of years, Jeff felt well enough intermittently for some travel and socializing, and we were able to maintain some semblance of our pre-cancer lives. However, in the months following the encephalitis and then the tracheotomy, Jeff only left home for doctor's appointments or walks around the neighborhood to move his body and soak in the sun. Visitors to our home were primarily limited to immediate family; our contact with the outside world was shrinking as the end drew close. Everything exhausted Jeff. Sitting in silence and napping for hours filled most of his days.

Jeff didn't have the energy, strength, or patience to make small talk; he was living with unbearable pain all day.

He was dying, and we couldn't stop it.

I watched as his eyes, once full of joy, slowly filled with disappointment and sadness. He knew he could no longer control the cancer taking over his body as it violently stole all pleasures from his life. He found no value or purpose in living most days. Our lives were filled with fear, isolation, and despair.

I didn't tell Jeff when I received invitations because I knew he would want me to go without him, but I wanted to stay and comfort him through his suffering. With his body rapidly declining, our time together was vanishing before our eyes. We were both trying to protect each other. I attempted to shield him from any misplaced guilt since his health was the reason for not going out. And he tried to make sure I was still enjoying life outside our home with family and friends, even though he couldn't. We both continuously thought of the other. I could see it in his eyes at times, and occasionally, he made a subtle comment that I was "missing out" on life, taking care of him.

I could only imagine the agony and conflicting thoughts he carried alone. Of course, I yearned for our life back—we both did—but I wanted to share the time we had with him. Nothing was the same without Jeff. I was madly in love with that man, and my heart was desperately attempting to capture moments to carry me through the inevitable dark days and nights I would soon face without him by my side. Jeff's body was not only visibly weakening physically, but I could also see his emotional and mental surrendering begin to take over. His once indestructible body of armor, which valiantly fought with steel strength and determination, was crumbling before my eyes. Cancer was slowly, steadily stealing the man I fell in love with in Vegas and shattering our hearts.

My parents lived twelve minutes from our home, and I knew Jeff was stable enough for me to leave for a handful of hours, so I decided to attend my parents' barbecue for a quick visit. I placed all of Jeff's pills on the kitchen island next to a big sheet of paper with handwritten instructions to remind him when to take each set in case I wasn't back in time for the next round of pills. I cleared the secretions and debris in his trach with a suction catheter. Then, I cleaned the trach machine, replaced the distilled water, and carefully replaced the dressings around the trach. I placed extra trach suctions, dressings, and towels nearby just in case he needed anything for those few hours when I was gone.

I carefully arranged the recently upped doses of fentanyl patches for the pain, along with the multiple daily doses of Norco, OxyContin, gabapentin, and dexamethasone. Those were the most essential medications, as they helped with the overall agony he endured each day. Even with all of the medications, it only scratched the surface to dull his intense pain. Before I left, I made Jeff his favorite smoothie; he drank two to three smoothies daily.

We had tried so many different foods and drinks for nutrients, most of which he could not stomach or swallow; there were only a handful of menu items left that he could consume. He loved my homemade banana bread fresh from the oven, warm mashed potatoes smothered in butter, and a Wendy's frozen chocolate frosty. They were simple for him to digest, easy to swallow, and soothing to his highly sensitive tongue and throat. These were the staples in our home.

He could only eat soft foods that didn't require chewing due to the sharp, stabbing pain in his teeth. He especially enjoyed frozen foods, which added a tiny bit of relief as they froze the pain in his mouth and felt soothing. The other staple in our home was the Smart & Final Neapolitan ice cream. That was the most popular item in our home, so I always had a large backup tub in the garage freezer. The frozen sensation helped to temporarily numb the pain the pills didn't attack in his face, teeth, and mouth as he slowly swirled the ice cream on his tongue until it melted.

Jeff's face and head were his most concentrated areas of discomfort. He described it as if every nerve on his face, inside his mouth, and in his teeth were all afflicted with sharp, piercing, constant pain, which often left him sitting for hours on the couch, unable to move, speak, eat, or drink. He would stoically sit on the sofa, either downstairs or in our oversized master bedroom chair, with his face lowered into both his hands while he was bent over, patiently praying the pain would dissipate.

I felt so helpless knowing we had just upped his pain medications at our weekly appointment, and the next appointment to assess his pain wasn't for a few days. The powerless feeling after years of watching my love continually deteriorate every minute of the day, with little I could do to take away his suffering, was defeating and debilitating to both our spirits. It was enough to destroy even the strongest person. I can recall many long days and endless nights writhing with overwhelming feelings of anxiety and inadequacy because I knew there was nothing I could do to lessen his pain. By that time, the only thing I could offer was the certainty that he knew I was by his side—that he was not alone in those dark hours—and that he could feel my unwavering, unbreakable love and support.

I had always been able to place fear on a shelf in the back corners of my mind. I became an expert at limiting the amount of time I spent in fear. I found ways to climb out of that despondent space and allow my resiliency and resolve to pull me into a position of strength. However, at times, I knew I needed to acknowledge the fear, cry with it, and even look ahead at my future fears—a life without my love. I could feel fear and desperation overpowering my strength as the months and weeks progressed.

That Father's Day, I was determined to keep fear far away. That day was about celebrating my wonderful dad and spending time with my circle of support—family and friends. Once Jeff put on a movie and was set up with everything he would need while I was gone, I leaned over and kissed him gently. Then I softly whispered, "Honey, I won't be gone long. Just a quick "Happy Father's Day" wish to Dad and a short visit, and I'll see you soon." He slowly placed his finger over the trach hole and wearily said, "Take your time, Honeybee. I'll be fine."

I could see his energy was already drained as he began to curl up on the couch for a long afternoon nap. I knew a slight diversion and change of scenery would benefit us both, reminding myself there was no reason to feel guilty because I knew I couldn't pour from an empty cup. When you're a long-term caregiver, it's easy to lose yourself. While it wasn't easy, I didn't allow guilt to creep in when I needed a break for self-care. I knew it was precisely what allowed me to sustain the intense pace for those three years. I learned to make guilt a fleeting thought, knowing that those breaks and moments of self-care were a vital part of our relationship in surviving that torturous battle with cancer.

Those first few minutes in the car after I left him home alone pained me as I so badly wanted Jeff to join me. I felt awful that I was able to leave home for a change of scenery and a reprieve from cancer, but his body gave him no respite. It always reminded him that he could never escape the mental and physical prison of his impending death.

I loved to spend time with my family and socialize with friends. However, when I was in town running errands and saw someone I knew, I would often turn and walk in the other direction. People thoughtfully asked for the most recent cancer update and how Jeff was doing; it was a prominent topic. We had lost so much of our identity during those years—we became the poster children for cancer, strength, and inspiration to others. I found so much comfort in all the community support surrounding us, but there were times we just wanted to escape it all. Everyone's intentions were always genuinely compassionate and concerned; they weren't doing anything wrong and meant no harm. People were worried and wanted to let me know they were thinking of and praying for us.

Our beautiful city of Chino Hills felt tiny everywhere I went. Having lived in the same city for twenty-five years and raising my children there, our roots and the tremendous support were strong. I didn't expect others to know that I wanted to escape talking about Jeff, his pain, and the latest tumors; I just wanted to grab a few groceries or gas. Intentions were noble, and I was grateful for all the heartfelt well wishes, but it was too overwhelming to constantly talk about Jeff's cancer and suffering everywhere I went.

I snuck into my parents' home like a stranger, hoping to go unnoticed. That day, I thought I could hug my dad and sit quietly with him alone for a few minutes. There was a part of me that had lost the ability to socialize; it felt insignificant to discuss everyday topics when Jeff was dying. Everything else felt inconsequential when we were barely hanging on to life as the inevitable end drew near.

When you're living through hell, small talk seems insignificant. I wasn't up to engaging in a dozen conversations, updating everyone on

Jeff and how I was holding up. I wanted to walk in and scream so loud that everyone could hear me all at once:

"Life is shitty; Jeff is dying a slow, painful death! I'm losing the love of my life; we're losing each other a little more every day! There are more tumors, more pain meds, and more treatments. I'm exhausted at every turn, and there is nothing remotely positive to share anymore; there's no more hope. Life Fucking Sucks!"

I'm sure everyone would have understood and given me the grace I desperately needed to relieve all my frustrations. But instead, I just quickly ran through my hellos to everyone to avoid a dramatic release of my extreme emotions.

All I wanted was to feel normal, but how could I when I had somehow lost my identity along the way? I had become a new version of myself, built for battle, not casual talk. *Would I ever find my old self again, or would this new version remain a part of me forever?* I wondered.

Everyone's face always did the same thing; it dropped down with their eyes as I could hear the pity and sadness in their hello. I wanted to have casual, everyday conversations, but I forgot how to. Maybe it was me; perhaps I changed into this new version that could only talk about Jeff and his cancer. I could hear the sharpness in my tone at inappropriate times that I couldn't control; everyone lovingly understood I wasn't my old cheerful self anymore.

Cancer had almost wholly consumed me over the past few years. As a caregiver, I often put my needs aside as I poured all my energy into saving Jeff. The unpredictability of cancer and the fear of losing him were always present, fostering irritability and irrational behavior at times. The burden of continuously making life-and-death decisions carried a heavy weight that almost broke me time and again. The painful reminders of the life we had lost and the anticipatory grief, knowing I would lose him one day, terrified me. My world was shrinking, with conversations centering around treatments and prognoses. Many people did not understand the emotional toll I was experiencing; I was losing my connection to the outside world. I thank God for the patience of my family and friends, who gave me the grace and space to accept the new (albeit temporary) version of myself without judgment, as I had become hyper-focused.

When your entire focus for three years is to save your loved one's life and ease their pain, the structural foundations of who you are shift subtly over time. The cancer had taken over who Jeff and I were as individuals. Jeff's calm, unassuming, and humble demeanor sometimes turned demanding, irritated, and indignant. Of course, his behavior and outlook on life would change; how could it not? Not everyone understood these shifts in us, and some of our relationships suffered. We became unapologetic as we fought to save his life.

That afternoon, I enjoyed my dad's flavorful barbecue strip steak marinated in lime, and his other secret seasonings that sizzled over his charcoal briquettes. I stayed for a couple of hours before it was time for me to find my way home. I was preparing to leave when Lorri, a family friend, tapped me on the shoulder. Lorri checked in with me weekly and sometimes daily. She always went out of her way to send me texts full of faith and hope; she was one of the many positive constants in my life with her genuinely kind support. Her thoughtful texts positively impacted both me and Jeff and lifted me out of many of the dark holes I fell into.

That afternoon at the barbecue, she offered me a warm embrace and asked if we could talk for a few minutes before I left. When she let go of the hug, I sensed something was different. Typically, she exudes a genuine warm radiance, but I sensed nervousness and anxiety that day. She wanted to go somewhere private to talk.

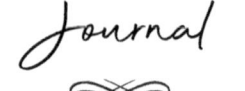

When we give so much of ourselves to care for someone we love, it can feel selfish to step away and tend to our own needs, but in truth, it's essential for survival. Think back to a time when you allowed yourself a moment of rest or joy in the middle of a heavy season. How did that choice affect your ability to show up for the people who needed you most?

Chapter 17

BACKYARD SECRETS

At Lorri's request to speak privately, I led her to a hidden corner of my parents' backyard. As we drew close, the overgrown eucalyptus trees swayed ominously in the cool summer breeze. Facing me, she took a few deep breaths, followed by an extensive pause. Tears welled up in her eyes when words finally began to form.

"I have prayed hard about this, and although it's against my religious beliefs, I need to share something with you. Have you heard of dying with dignity?"

My body tensed up and froze as tears started to pour out of me quickly. A few silent minutes passed with us both in tears, holding each other's hands.

Finally, I asked, "I'm sorry, what did you say?"

Not only is my friend one of the gentlest and most caring individuals I have ever known, but she is a very devout Christian. The conversation was a walking contradiction. Not only had the thought never crossed my mind, but she was the last person I could have ever imagined would bring it up.

I couldn't absorb what I had just heard. My thoughts started to spiral out of control. My heart was even further behind. *Is this even legal in California?* I thought. Was she talking about Dr. Kevorkian, euthanasia?

"Dr. Death" was the nickname given to Dr. Jack Kevorkian in the 1980s and 1990s. I recalled a class I took at UCLA where the concept of euthanasia was discussed. At the time, it was considered radical and highly controversial. In that class, we debated both sides of the delicate, vital, and unfortunately taboo topic: Should euthanasia be legalized in the U.S.? Was the act of taking one's life considered compassion or murder?

During that time, my brother was battling cancer, and I remember debating the subject in class at twenty years old. At the time, I thought, *Would this be something my brother could consider one day? Is it a selfish or selfless act of the patient and the caregiver? How does one choose between the struggle of selfishly never wanting to lose a loved one and, at the same time, wanting them to be free from the bondage of excruciating suffering?*

The last time I could recall hearing anything on the subject of dying with dignity was in 2014 when I read about a young woman, Brittany Maynard, who was dying a slow and painful death from cancer. She moved with her family to Oregon, where dying with dignity was legal. Until that very moment, sitting in my parents' peaceful backyard, I thought Oregon was the only state in the U.S. where it was legal to end a loved one's suffering compassionately.

My focus suddenly centered back on what Lorri shared with me, and my mind raced back to Jeff. We'd spent the first few years as a couple carefully and strategically planning our lives together so we could live in the same country. But these past few years, our sole focus had become aggressively advocating to save his life. What my friend was proposing was to end it all, to end our life together. Her intentions were compassionate and pure, and her only motive was to offer me a solution to end Jeff's suffering.

She knew Jeff lived every hour in horrific pain and that his deterioration was moving at a fast pace. Knowing what a devout Christian she is, I knew it was against her belief system, which made her approaching me with the idea of dying with dignity even more powerful. I knew the act of ending one's life of suffering was something she would never do. Her courage and compassion to set her beliefs aside to offer Jeff liberation from the excruciating pain was an incredibly selfless act.

Lorri had learned about dying with dignity from a friend of hers named Angie, who chose to assist her husband in the process. With tears streaming down her face, Lorri shared Angie and Frank's story with me. They'd had a similar experience with Frank's cancer and chose to end his life compassionately at home. The couple were also devout Christians, and other than Lorri, they told no one what they had done out of fear they'd be judged. They had struggled with their religious beliefs amidst the staggering pain Frank endured.

Lorri shared their story with me because she sensed our story was painfully similar. She didn't want Jeff to continue suffering needlessly, knowing it was terminal, and we were running out of options and hope. The common threads were mercy and compassion. The sympathy and kindness in my friend's eyes spoke volumes. She was a merciful angel delivering a message of hope to end Jeff's suffering.

I listened to her explain what Angie and Frank had done to end Frank's life, and once again, I could hear that unwelcome clock swiftly ticking at a pace we couldn't slow down. I knew nothing could prevent or delay the inevitable outcome. Jeff and I knew it was getting closer each day, and our endless marathon was nearing its final lap.

How could I allow myself to consider even the thought of us choosing to end his life, though? I wondered.

I wanted to run in the other direction, far away from the conversation. My focus for the past three years had been finding a cure, saving Jeff's life, and buying more time.

Could this be where we're at now? Would we need to take his life to end his suffering? I wondered.

In hindsight, hearing this from my devout Christian friend wasn't such a contradiction. She was a compassionate individual who loved us both immensely, and she knew the extreme torture Jeff's body was enduring relentlessly each day. I was stretched to my limits daily, and I could see Jeff's pain threshold decreasing rapidly. As the intensity of pain increased, his tolerance and patience decreased, and more anger set in. His will to fight and live were noticeably waning.

But how was I supposed to say to the man I loved with every ounce of my soul that we had a choice to take control and end his suffering and pain? How could I find the words to share with him what I now knew? We knew we were losing the war, but neither dared to say it out loud. Jeff had fought so bravely with immeasurable fortitude and courage. Was it time to offer him the choice to die compassionately with dignity and stop his endless suffering?

Crippled by the weight of death in the quiet corner of my parent's backyard, I had a thousand torturous questions. The world whispered to the other guests promises of hope and summer dreams to come. They all chattered excitedly, of warm vacations and happy tidings, while I stood paralyzed by heartache and fear, unable to speak.

After a long stretch of heavy silence and more tears, I held Lorri tightly and thanked her for bravely sharing honestly with me. I'd been there too long and needed to leave my parents' home to process what I'd just learned. I quickly said goodbye to everyone and decided to drive a long detour home to buy some time to compose myself. I wandered through back roads into rolling hills as the sun set, and the indigo summer sky gave way to evening stars. On that drive, I found space to wander into our lives before cancer.

My mind drifted to a memorable Christmas season when I visited Jeff in Canada.

We drove to Calgary for a few days to enjoy the holiday festivities and stayed at the Fairmont Hotel. It was decorated beautifully with holiday lights, and the smell of fresh pine wreaths drifted around every corner, accented with the warm scents of nutmeg and cinnamon. Jeff and I soaked in the ambiance as we sat by the crackling fireplaces on our romantic holiday weekend.

We finished an elegant dinner the evening before I would fly back home, and the usual melancholy came over us both, knowing it would be weeks before we touched again. Walking toward an elevator, we noticed a line forming. Curious, we walked over to ask what the line was for and were told the group was heading into the Toyota holiday party. When we entered the elevator to our room, Jeff and I looked at each other and said, "Let's go to the party." We instantly went from sad to giddy as we went through our suitcases and changed into more appropriate clothes for a holiday party.

All freshened up and back downstairs, we nonchalantly joined the party line and acted like we belonged. Before we knew it, we were in. The somber night had turned into one of our most celebrated memories—a night of lively music, dancing, and making new friends. When people asked us what department we were in with Toyota, I naturally said I was in the legal department, and Jeff said he was in sales. We playfully sold our story to everyone that night as we shared cocktails, the dance floor, and laughter, losing ourselves in the festivities.

We requested a few songs at the DJ booth to bring the dance floor to life. After our arms and hands raised the roof into the early morning hours, we said our goodbyes to our new friends, who insisted we take some of the centerpieces and that they would see us next week at work. We obliged and laughed hysterically back to our room, carrying the large floral arrangements. Neither of us had ever crashed a party, but we both got so caught up in the spontaneity of the moment that we just went with it. Jeff and I played off each other in all facets of life. To this day, that holiday party remains one of my cherished memories, always bringing a smile to my heart and a youthful giggle. I'm constantly reminded how together we felt invincible.

Now, we were vulnerable and weak. Cancer had changed us. Together, we feared death and a life without the other. I sat silently in the garage for thirty minutes, contemplating what to do with the information I learned that day at the barbecue. I stepped through the door slowly, my shoulders heavy with the weight of the day. I saw Jeff peacefully watching a show while waiting for me.

He smiled and turned my way. "Hi Honeybee, how was your time with your dad?"

I'd drained all my tears in the car and was convincingly calm as I said with a forced smile, "Everyone says hi and asks about you, and they all send their love."

I looked over the medications to make sure no pills were missed, and then I prepared for the evening. I repeated the same routine I had done before I left, from cleaning the trach and the dressings to putting on hospital gloves and replacing the fentanyl patches. Then, we made our way upstairs for an early night.

We lay in bed, holding hands like every night. Jeff fell asleep first, which gave me the space I needed to continue processing. That was one of the only times I appreciated Jeff's hearing loss, an impairment caused by all the treatments. Thankfully, he didn't sleep with his hearing aids in, so I could take the time to hold him and softly weep without waking him.

I looked around the room as we lay in our cozy king bed covered in layers of crisp, white sheets and a soft, silver-toned down comforter draped gently over us. Serenity set in as I remembered how we chose the bedding and draperies together, as we had most things in our home. We enjoyed those mundane, everyday tasks, hand-picking the fabrics of our life hand in hand and creating the backdrop for our love story. Deep into the night, I considered our life together and the days gone by. Sometime in the wee hours of the morning, I fell into a fitful slumber. I wasn't ready to share what I had learned with Jeff; I needed more time to process the shock. Days passed while I kept the knowledge to myself. During that time, I struggled internally, secretly hoping and praying once again that God would be merciful and take away Jeff's agony.

The next few days were spent researching as much as I could get my hands on. My clinical side kicked in again, and I pushed aside my emotions. I dove deep into exploring our options and detached myself from the weight of the emotional burden on my shoulders. I welcomed the distraction until I could find the courage to look my love in the eyes and talk to him about dying. Up until then, our entire purpose had been living, looking for a cure or a plan to attack the latest tumors. I didn't know how to shift gears and create an open dialogue to discuss ending his life.

I needed to find the strength to force myself to broach the seemingly impossible subject. Once I had the information, I couldn't ignore it; I had to find a way to tell Jeff that I learned dying with dignity was legal in California. It became law in 2018, the same year Jeff was diagnosed.

As of 2024, dying with dignity is legal in ten states and a federal district (California, Oregon, Hawaii, Washington, Colorado, Montana, New Jersey, New Mexico, Maine, Vermont, and the District of Columbia), with several other states in the U.S. considering this legislation. I have learned since that day that there's a lack of awareness on the subject matter. I've also discovered that most people who perform the act choose not to discuss it or share their experiences. It's understandable why there is little discussion surrounding dying with dignity, as it's a very private, personal, and painful decision. However, keeping it contained makes the knowledge and awareness less accessible for those who need it most. It was heartbreaking to learn that many people are unaware it's an option for their loved one's needless suffering.

Friday, June 25, 2021, was the day I finally found the courage to discuss dying with dignity. Jeff was sitting downstairs on the couch with his legs elevated to alleviate the swelling in his lower extremities. The kids affectionately called Jeff's legs "chicken legs" because they were long and thin. Following cancer and all the treatments and medications, they had become so swollen that his socks left prominent indentations. The swelling wasn't contained just to his legs; it was everywhere; his stomach and face were the most noticeable. The body transformation hid the once-chiseled chest and narrow face with distinctive jaw lines and a chin dimple.

Finding the right words to talk to Jeff about dying still seemed impossible. There was no easy way to say it. Sitting beside him on the couch, I opened my mouth to let the words find their way out.

"Honey, I had an interesting talk with someone at the barbecue at my parents' home the other day."

He peacefully listened, utterly unaware of what I was going to share.

"Honey, Lorri took me aside and told me about one of her friends whose husband was suffering from cancer, and he, too, was in unbearable pain every day."

He innocently asked me what Lorri's friends did to relieve the horrific pain. I had to spit the words out and rip off that band-aid quickly.

"Honey, did you know it's legal in California to choose to end your life and die with dignity to stop your suffering? We have choices. You don't have to suffer like an animal dying in the woods waiting for the end to come."

A deep and crushing silence bore down and filled the room as tears flooded my vision and Jeff's face. I couldn't hold back the floodgates any longer, and I could see he was there too.

After the words left my mouth, it was as if a vacuum sucked all the air out of the room, and silence hung heavy. I cried, "Honey, I don't want you ever to leave me. I can't imagine one minute without you, but I see the torturous pain you're in daily, and we can't ease your suffering. This may be something we want to look into."

We wept and held each other like so many times before. When the tears slowed down, he placed his finger on the trach hole, and at that moment, I could see this thought was not a new one to him.

With his medical background, he had already contemplated options he hadn't yet shared with me. What I didn't know is that our minds were independently coming to the same conclusion, as the suffering was intensifying each week. By that time, the unwelcome traveler had robbed Jeff of all his dignity; it was only a matter of time before it took his life. Although there were no immediate signs of his body shutting down on its own, we both knew the excruciating pain was becoming more than he could endure.

He looked at me and softly said between tears and breaths, "Yes, I know this is an option."

No more words were spoken until a few weeks later, when we made the appointment with our doctors to begin the process.

Our hearts and souls were broken. Cancer had stripped and transformed us both into unrecognizable versions of ourselves. Living a life with no quality was not a life Jeff wanted to live. There was no more hope, and now his only purpose in living had become waiting to die as he suffered in an endless nightmare of excruciating pain.

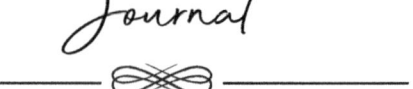

Some conversations change us forever, opening a door to thoughts and choices we never imagined we'd have to face. Take a quiet moment to reflect on a time when someone's honesty, however difficult, shifted your perspective. How did that moment shape the way you approached the days or decisions that followed?

Chapter 18
THE FINAL RING

We couldn't imagine an hour without each other, but our focus shifted. Somehow, we needed to find a way to accept our new path and end Jeff's pain. My mind had to start processing and envisioning a life without my love. By that stage, everything in our lives felt like a nightmare we would never wake up from.

Slowly and painfully, our hearts were forced to acknowledge the reality of what was soon to occur. We were entering unknown territory; no one we knew had gone through the process of dying with dignity. We could find very little information on the subject, and once again, we felt frightened and isolated. Although it was legal in California, no one we spoke with knew it was a legal option other than our doctors. Dying with dignity was seemingly an unspoken subject matter. Like the past three years, we navigated another unfamiliar, clearly defined, and terrifying fork in the road.

With his decline progressing rapidly, Jeff had to decide before the choice was no longer his to make—before his body or mind betrayed him completely. We didn't know exactly how much time we had; we might have had two months, but we knew his abilities could shift in an instant, leaving Jeff trapped without options. The sand in the hourglass was nearly gone, each grain slipping through faster than we could grasp, a silent reminder that time was running out.

He could continue to live with relentlessly excruciating pain and no quality of life, or we could start down a path of choosing to end his suffering. Soon, I would no longer be able to care for him. Once he became mentally incapacitated and could no longer feed himself, he would lose the power to choose to die with dignity at home, as these are two of the legal requirements. Living on life support or lying in a bed, unable to function on his own, was not a life Jeff wanted. He made it painfully clear he would never put himself or me through that.

Jeff existed, but he was no longer living.

It would take time to absorb the harshness of our remaining choices, and whether we would move forward in choosing death with dignity as our path. It was by far the most earth-shattering and heartbreaking decision of our lives. All the possibilities we were forced to envision left us frozen in fear. We spent days ruminating on how one chooses their last day, last breath, last good morning and goodnight, and their last "I love you." Most days, it was more than our minds and hearts could process. However, allowing Jeff to be tortured with pain as he suffered silently, with no end in sight, felt equally paralyzing.

We began coming to terms with fully surrendering our will to fight in order to create a peaceful ending. The end was fast approaching like a runaway train; there was no way to slow down the cancer or Jeff's inevitable end. I forced my mind to accept a life without him while concurrently soaking in every last scent and touch. Slowly, I acknowledged and resigned myself to the horror before us.

Jeff and I had spent several days painfully discussing whether dying at home with dignity was an option for us—whether it would be something we could accept in our situation. We could feel the weight in each conversation as our minds struggled to form words that focused on his final day. It was agonizing to look at the man who held my entire heart and imagine myself handing him a concoction that would stop his. Each of those discussions left me both detaching myself from him for self-preservation and simultaneously holding on with all my strength. We knew logically the most compassionate solution was to allow him to die peacefully at home. However, allowing logic to prevail over our emotions tested our mental courage and love for each other in profound ways, as we were about to look death head-on voluntarily. By the end of those several days, we'd made a decision despite our inability to fathom the reality.

The following week, we had an appointment at City of Hope. It was then that we first cautiously discussed dying with dignity with our doctors.

We had several appointments scheduled for one day and held firmly onto each other as we sat through each. That day, the rooms felt smaller than usual. My mouth was dry and my throat was tight, but we finally found the courage to speak to our doctors about what we'd been contemplating. The soft, beige leather and cloth chairs felt sterile and cold as we sat with each doctor in the stark white rooms. First, we met with our medical oncologist, then our radiation oncologist, and finally, our pain management team. Forming the words never got easier as tears gently rolled down my cheeks. Instead of discussing medical options or more pain medications, as we had the past few years, that day, we informed our doctors that we were there to discuss Jeff's death.

Despite the coolness of the rooms, I could feel heat radiating from my entire body. My heart pounded, and my body tensed up, knowing what we were there to ask for. I memorized every detail of each doctor's appearance, the sound of their voices, and the details of the rooms, and I hung onto each word they spoke, knowing our time with them was coming to an end. My mind captured the last memories of the team and hospital that soon would no longer be an integral part of our lives. The world felt deathly silent as I forced myself to bring up dying with dignity.

Tentatively, taking long, deep breaths, I somehow forced out the words hidden in the furthest parts of my mind. Expecting a negative response from the doctors who had fought so hard to save Jeff, I waited for them to try to talk us out of it or be disappointed in our decision. Instead, as I spoke the words, "We want to know what our options might be regarding dying with dignity," I saw compassion in their eyes and a calmness in their demeanor. Their consistent reactions lent an unexpected amount of comfort and peace to each room. I could feel each doctor's sincere sympathy as we faced a horrifying decision and prepared to end the torturous pain Jeff was enduring.

Our doctors freely shared their views on the subject and their insight on whether it was a viable option for Jeff. We didn't know what to expect or what their reaction might be, but to our surprise, our doctors fully supported our decision. Our last treatment was not far away, and no more hope remained. Jeff would be in hospice care soon, waiting to die while his body was slowly and painfully shutting down.

That day, we asked our doctors to begin putting everything in motion so that death with dignity could be an option for us. The guidelines and steps one has to take to qualify for dying with dignity are extensive. It may not be an option for everyone and should not be taken lightly. Several safeguards are in place to ensure this option is used with the utmost care and discretion.

We met each requirement for the end-of-life option: Jeff was over eighteen and terminally ill, and although we had beaten our original diagnosis, he was now without any more options. His life expectancy was less than the six months required, he independently and voluntarily requested the prescription for the medication from our physicians, and we attended multiple mental health specialist appointments addressing Jeff's medical history and his current physical and psychological state. The patient must have the mental capacity to make decisions, and they must be capable of self-administering and ingesting medications without assistance.

The only requirements that would likely one day change due to the continually spreading cancer were if he could no longer administer the drugs or if his mental faculties deteriorated. There were occasional, momentary shifts in his mental capacity, and having the cognitive capabilities to make that crucial decision was imperative. One time, I found Jeff in the middle of the night in his pajamas, pulling the car out of the garage to "pick up Maddie from the airport." He believed she was waiting for him.

It was a delicate balance to convince him to come back inside so he didn't make that long, dangerous drive in the middle of the night while he was on so many narcotics. At that point, I began to hide all the car keys. He was also haphazardly moving money from our bank accounts, so I had to lock him out of the accounts to keep our finances intact. It was heartbreaking to take away more of his dignity, which added additional stress to our relationship, but I had no other choice. These incidents only happened intermittently, but they were serious. I could see his mental capacity declining as the destructive cancer and pain medications affected his cognitive ability at times.

We planned our strategy for saving Jeff's life from the first diagnosis, so it seemed appropriate that we would now direct the journey on how he would die. The next step was receiving the prescription from our doctor, which is not covered by insurance; it's done through a private company. We followed each step methodically and tried our best not to think of the implications of our actions. We needed to stay as clinical as possible and try to keep our emotions at bay. Once he was deemed qualified for the end-of-life option and the medications were ordered, all that was left to do was wait.

In early August, there was an unexpected ring at my front door. When I answered it, a stranger stood on the stoop holding a brown paper bag with red tape across the top. I knew immediately who the man was and what he was bringing into our home. I wanted to be polite and thank him, but I couldn't form words for the unfortunate delivery driver bringing the deadly dose of drugs into our home. Instead, I abruptly grabbed the bag from him and panicked; I didn't know what to do with it.

Frantically shutting the door, I ran around, trying to figure out where to hide the small bag of opioids that was filled with heavy doses of peace and sorrow. I didn't want to hold it or have it in our home; I wanted to put it in a place I could avoid. I hoped hiding it would blind me to the reminders that came with it. I hurriedly placed the bag in the pantry, hidden in the back corner of the kitchen. I found large pantry items high on a shelf to tuck the bag behind. There, carefully concealed, I could avoid it and pretend the brown bag and its frightening contents didn't exist.

At the time, our fifty-third birthdays were approaching, which normally meant preparing for fun celebrations. Every year, I looked forward to my birthday for weeks before it arrived. But that birthday was drastically different. It was impossible to feel joyous or festive as an impenetrable dark cloud loomed over our every waking moment. A heavy weight bore down on me as the large, ominous shadow of death left no openings for light to enter. Our home had become a place I barely recognized. Not just aesthetically, with all the medical supplies, devices, and medications, but our home had become vacant of laughter and hope. It was overshadowed by sorrow and fear that occupied every nook and cranny, creeping into every fiber of our beings and crippling us.

We didn't know when Jeff's last breath would be, but we knew he wouldn't see another year begin. Over the past several months, as his health diminished exponentially, that was one thing we could see clearly through the darkness. We knew we would not grow old together, and time would soon stand still for Jeff.

Acknowledging the future we would never see was an essential part of the ongoing grieving process. We had to accept and somehow embrace our bleak and brutal reality. Instead of planning barbecues and travel, we planned who would lead his "Celebration of Love" services in Canada and California and what he wanted them to look and feel like. Every conversation was crushing as we went over the details of his eventual demise.

We discussed his wishes for cremation and where he wanted his ashes spread at the family farm in Canada and a few other special places. Most days, our conversations centered around death; it seemed impossible to escape. Following discussions with our doctors, it was decided that there would be one last set of radiation treatments before putting Jeff in hospice and ending our care at City of Hope. We were out of options as the cancer was floating in his spinal fluid and brain. There were limits to how much more they could radiate before risking irreversible spinal paralysis or brain damage. Medically, there was nothing more to be done after this next set of radiation treatments.

The day had arrived for our last appointment at City of Hope. Waking up on that sweltering August day, the sun shone so strongly that you could feel it piercing your skin. We were withdrawn in our home as we quietly got ready, with no conversation. It was an eerie feeling, similar to preparing to attend a funeral. Our once-vibrant home felt somber. We went through the motions, showering and getting dressed in a haze of disbelief. Grief consumed us, and the air carried a very real and palpable weight. The deafening silence in our home was punctuated by the familiar sounds of running water and cabinets closing as we prepared to leave. These familiar sounds seemed louder than usual; everything felt quiet yet exaggerated. We were suspended between the past, the present, and Jeff's looming death. We knew with certainty that after that day, death was unavoidable. We could feel the momentum of the unstoppable power as death cruelly came for Jeff.

Having driven thousands of miles over the course of three years to our home away from home, we were on autopilot as I drove us onto the 210 freeway alongside the beautiful foothills and the ominous mountains that led the way to the hospital. On our countless car rides those past three years, there was always a sense of hope and something to fight for, even if it was slight. But on that last day, our spirits were broken, and our heads hung low. Defeat lay heavy upon each of us.

Exiting the freeway, I saw the tall buildings enclosing the enormous hospital campus. We passed the new building that began construction earlier that year, the Hope Village Hotel for patients and their families.

With no plans to return, we knew we would never see the new hotel completed. Everything we saw on that trip would be the last we saw of City of Hope.

We turned onto the tree-lined, lengthy front driveway entrance and parked the car. Slowly, we walked past the koi ponds and City of Hope's wishing tree, which displays patients' and their families' notes of healing and hope. Finally, we made our way past the rose garden, where I had spent countless days alone praying to God and pondering what our lives and future may look like. During all those years, I never once thought about what our last visit to the hospital would look like.

For many patients, the last visit means they're cured. They can go home, enjoy family, and plan for the future. But for me and Jeff, that last visit to the hospital meant it was the end. There was nothing more our team of doctors could do; we had exhausted everything, and all hope and time would elude us.

City of Hope is one of only fifty-six National Cancer Institute-designated comprehensive cancer centers in the U.S. Their credo is, "There is no profit in curing the body if, in the process, we destroy the soul." I had read those words, which were inscribed in the rose garden, many times before; they were powerful and accurate. Over those years, we'd struggled countless times with this principle. *How far do we push modern medicine or Jeff's body?* It became a delicate balance of fighting for more time and weighing that against the quality of Jeff's life as it deteriorated. Deep down, in the places we never brought to the surface, we knew Jeff's last day would find us eventually, and that day had suddenly arrived.

City of Hope was a beacon of light for us. With every visit, we felt blessed and reassured by everyone at that facility, who cared for Jeff with precise knowledge and loving grace while continually helping us find hope and maintain dignity. Entering the building for the last time, we walked down the hallway to the elevator, which took us to the basement floor where the radiation department was located.

Jeff and I walked in silence, holding hands firmly, our bodies tense. Without a word, we could sense each other's fear, unspoken but undeniable. We were taking our final lap in the cancer marathon, our hearts racing with despair and anxiety, knowing we would never take that walk again. Slowly stepping out of the elevator, I checked Jeff in and let the staff know we had arrived for Jeff's last treatment; I could feel the bitterness of those words roll off my tongue as I held back tears.

Jeff and I sat in the waiting room in silence.

There was no small talk, no words to comfort each other.

Knowing it was our last radiation treatment filled me with contradicting emotions. Jeff would never have needles poking him again or have to spend hours preparing for and going through all the scans, custom-made masks, and the litany of doctors' visits.

It was all ending; there was no more hope.

Once the hospital released us, Jeff would be in hospice, something we both were well aware was the final stage of at-home care before death. We sat quietly waiting, nerves and anxieties building as we held hands tightly. I could feel the sweat in our restless palms and could see the despondency in Jeff's eyes. Sitting still in that nightmare moment felt surreal. "Jeff Dunphy," the nurses called out. My heart raced, but I sat frozen next to Jeff, neither of us moving. We looked into each other's eyes, devastated, trying not to lose our shit right there in the middle of the waiting room. Everyone around us was optimistically awaiting their turn to be called in for their radiation appointment, their eyes and hearts still full of hope. They still had a fight and choices that Jeff no longer had. Soon, Jeff's body would begin to lose its ability to operate as the cancer further infiltrated his spine, which controlled so much of his body's ability to function.

A tight ball once again rose in my throat, and neither of us could hold back the tears any longer. "Jeff Dunphy," they called again. We both wiped away tears and put on stoic faces, holding hands with an intense grip. That grip spoke volumes of the melancholy our voices could not speak in that silent waiting room.

This is it. The long, hard-fought, heroic battle was over. Together, side by side, we valiantly attacked every tumor and faced every surgery, radiation, and chemo treatment. We had courageously and methodically created a strategy to buy more time and were temporarily successful, but that time was now up.

Over the past several months, we came to realize that there was no more quality time to buy. We were destroying Jeff's soul, and there was no cure. There was nothing more for Jeff to gain. God and Jeff's body were letting us know he'd had enough. We needed to begin to let go. "Jeff Dunphy?" they called a third time.

We lifted each other out of our chairs and held each other steady as we walked together, for the last time, down the hallway toward the radiation room. When we entered the room, I felt as though we were laying down our metaphorical swords and surrendering. The mood in the room was drastically different on that day. We weren't trying to kill the newest tumors; we were trying to radiate certain tumors in his brain for a second time, and the entire spine would be receiving radiation.

The purpose of that last radiation series was to kill everything the scans displayed and anything we couldn't see in those scans. Once fully radiated, no more treatments could be performed on that region again. It was being done in an effort to hold back the effects of the innumerable tumors that were attempting to control his spine. Jeff's last treatment would not give us more time to live and enjoy life, but rather, it would provide us with a brief period before he would no longer be able to function on his own.

We knew the tumors were beginning to invade parts of the spine that would affect Jeff's ability to function. We could only hold them at bay for so long until they would begin to take over Jeff's speech and ability to walk, drink, eat, and use the restroom without assistance. Jeff absolutely refused to live on those terms, which he'd made abundantly clear. He didn't want to be trapped alive, left only to breathe. His life had been full of purpose and laughter. Lying unconscious in a hospital bed was not an option for Jeff. He would not allow that.

I walked up to Jeff before they placed and tightened the mask on his head. We usually said a prayer together and prayed that the radiation would eradicate all the tumors and help buy us time to be together to find a cure. That prayer no longer applied. Instead, we softly told each other how much we loved each other and prayed for peace in our hearts as tears streamed heavily down our cheeks. I kissed him gently like I did before every treatment and sullenly walked out of the room, feeling lost and defeated.

I couldn't imagine what my love was deliberating, the fear that he must have experienced, strapped in that mask while the radiation targeted the tumors in his spine and brain. The emotional scars of hundreds of radiation treatments endured over the years were deeply rooted; those scars were permanent. He must have felt terror and isolation during every treatment, but especially that day as he lay still on that cold, hard table that moved him into the tunnel that no longer promised more life. It was a sick feeling, knowing that it was his last treatment and only death awaited him on the other side.

Overwhelmed with the knowledge of what Jeff was going through, I made my way to a quiet corner where I could be alone to let the pain out as I cried and prayed to God desperately for mercy. The strength Jeff exemplified during his three and a half years of cancer treatment was extraordinary. The fight he put in every minute of every day was purely heroic. Meditating on all those things that day, my heart was broken. Despite his best efforts, there was no way to stop what was certain to come next.

When Jeff came out of the radiation room with the usual indentations on his face from the mask, I forced out an insincere smile as I said, "That's it, honey, we're all done."

We both knew there was nothing to celebrate. We tried our best, and the nurses and reception staff all came out to congratulate Jeff as they always did when he finished a radiation series. *Did they all know it was his last treatment ever? Did they know Jeff would die soon? Would they be clapping and congratulating us if they knew?*

They had the best intentions as they handed Jeff his umpteenth medal and certificate of completion while he resentfully rang the bell to signal it was his last treatment to everyone in the waiting room. Usually, after ringing the bell, we'd find our way home to celebrate the two months of freedom that lay ahead before the next scan. *Would there even be two months left together?* I reflected with a heavy heart. That day, the sound of the bell was drastically different than before. Instead of hopeful, it sounded ominous, bringing a sense of foreboding and despair into our hearts and piercing our souls like daggers.

Following the radiation treatment, we went over for our last visit with Dr. Amini, a young, unassuming groom-to-be with thick, black hair. He dressed professionally for every appointment in a suit, dress shirt, and tie, and always wore a large, friendly smile under his warm, compassionate eyes. Over our countless visits, we'd learned much about the distinguished doctor. We knew he was to be married that fall, so we congratulated him on finding love and the person he wanted to spend the rest of his life with, one of life's greatest gifts. We also learned the date of his birthday, which was only days before mine.

Over the years, Dr. Amini added special touches to our medical journey, such as giving us his cell phone number so we could contact him directly if we needed anything. On those rare occasions when I texted him, he wrote back instantly, ready to assist us as if we were his only patients. He extended himself far beyond our expectations and exemplified every outstanding quality a doctor can possess. Dr. Amini became an integral part of our extraordinary journey.

That afternoon, August 16, 2021, we patiently waited in the room to see Dr. Amini for our last visit. As we sat side by side, holding each other, the anxiety began to build. The waiting seemed to take longer than usual because we were so antsy that day. Finally, he and his staff walked in, a larger group than normal. Usually it was just the doctor, but a handful of nurses and other reception staff joined him in the room that day.

They walked in carrying white-on-white cupcakes (my favorite) and candles as they sang "Happy Birthday" to me in beautiful unison while one of the nurses videotaped. Jeff and I were amazed at the thoughtfulness, how the doctor remembered it was my birthday, and that white buttercream icing on white cake was my favorite. To say he went above and beyond for us over the years would be a vast understatement. For the first time that day, Dr. Amini and his staff helped Jeff and I find our smiles. It felt like it had been days since any feeling of joy had washed over us.

Trying to make the moment last as long as possible, we all chatted about anything to fill the time, and then we took a few pictures with Dr. Amini. We were in no hurry because we knew when we left, the team that had worked so hard for years to buy us time would no longer be a part of our lives. Dr. Amini had other patients; it was time for our final goodbyes. Jeff leaned in first, and they hugged for a long time as Jeff tried to gently speak words of gratitude through the trach and the tears. When it was my turn, I held onto him like he was family. I didn't know how to thank him for all he had done for us.

That day, we were filled with admiration, friendship, gratitude, and great sadness, knowing we would never see him again. There was no shortage of tears in the room. Before leaving, I realized that I felt lost.

What were we supposed to do next? Who would I call if I needed help? Did we simply wait for Jeff to die? Or did we open that brown bag? My mind anxiously wondered.

So many horrifying thoughts entered my mind. *What would happen when the tumors began to take over the essential functions of Jeff's body, and he could no longer walk, talk, use the restroom, bathe himself, or feed himself? Would I need to move him into a facility one day if I could no longer take care of him myself? Would it get to that point?*

We walked out of the room filled with warm, loving hearts and into the cold hospital corridors. Back outside in the warm California sun, there was not enough summer heat to take away the chill in our hearts.

For the first time in my life, I dreaded my birthday the following day. I couldn't shake the trepidation that consumed me. I knew my life was about to start over without Jeff in it. I had been living in the present since the day I met Jeff, soaking in every ounce of the energy that our love brought into my life. But as we left City of Hope behind that day, I could feel my heart begin to let go of us slowly, and I started to agonize over what my tomorrows would be like without him. It wasn't the first time I had allowed my mind to wander there, but it was the first time it felt tangible and real, a future that I could no longer avoid. Shortly, I would have to learn how to live my life alone without Jeff. To wake up each day without his touch, without his practical jokes that made me laugh until my cheeks hurt. Soon, I would never again hear the sound of his loving voice calling me "Honeybee." Whose hand would I reach for to hold on every car drive?

In the years since our engagement, we had planned and put together lists for our wedding. We relished the thought of what that day would look like as we planned all the tiny details of how we would celebrate our love with the special people in our lives surrounding us. We made a guest list and music playlist, curated venue options, and put together many other splendid wedding details. Jeff even loved to look at dresses with me, never short on compliments of how he envisioned me walking down the aisle one day, saying how breathtaking I would look as I approached him. But the wedding never took place.

We had every intention to say our vows and formally commit to each other for the rest of our lives in front of our family and friends. However, after the cancer diagnosis, we thought about it now and then, but in the chaos of treatments, it never became a top priority. For me and Jeff, there was no doubt that we were committed to each other. It was forever, a once-in-a-lifetime love, and we knew that a piece of paper would not change our dedication, even though we yearned for that day. I don't recall who said it first or the day it started, but we called each other "husband and wife;" we had an unbreakable bond and didn't need the formal paper to remind us.

Jeff was up well before me when I awoke to the start of my fifty-third year. He made sure I didn't venture downstairs until he was ready. I could hear a subtle lightness in his voice, asking me to wait a bit longer to head down for coffee. Finally, I got the go-ahead and was warmly welcomed by streamers, balloons, and decorations in my favorite blue colors. With the assistance of his sister and brother-in-law, Jeff had been determined to make my last birthday with him unforgettable. They opened the large glass door panels accordioned into each other, opening to the backyard patio. The fountains were running as the pool glistened in the morning sun. A backdrop of majestic mountains stood tall as the warm summer breeze wafted into the room. For the first time in months, our home felt like "our home." There were glimpses of the love, joy, laughter, and music it once held.

Jeff must have been collecting this energy for weeks. I don't know how he could have possibly gathered the strength to help everyone plan such a beautiful celebration, but it meant the world to me. Knowing it would likely be a short-lived burst of energy, we savored each second, allowing ourselves to get lost in those few hours blissfully. I never saw that part of Jeff again; he pushed himself too far that day for me, but those beautiful memories are forever locked away.

He'd left a beautiful love note on the coffee maker for me that morning, yet another reminder of his love and devotion.

"With you, God wished me, my ANGEL ... Always to be with me, Never far away, Giving a heart like no other, Even with a broken heart, Life that only others dream."

With his unsteady, trembling hands, he formed each shaky letter. Every word showed the tremendous effort and strength it took him to write that love letter for me. After seven and a half years, with thousands of love notes and cards, even with all his body had endured, Jeff always found a new, beautiful way to say "I love you." There were no unspoken words left between us, and I am eternally grateful for that gift we gave each other. He wanted to leave me with a lasting memory on my birthday, and he did just that. He was dying, but we never stopped living for each other.

Exerting so much of himself, he was depleted of energy shortly after breakfast and needed to go upstairs to rest for the remainder of the day. Later that evening, following a long rest, Jeff placed a gift next to the white-on-white buttercream cake as we blew out the last birthday candles we would ever share together.

Handing me the gift, Jeff tenderly said, "You should have gotten this long ago."

Inside the box was a beautiful wedding band embedded with a row of diamonds. It was engraved with "A&F, Honeybee." Placing the wedding band next to my engagement ring, I wept uncontrollably as I tried to find a way to extend the day. I desperately wanted time to stop. The guttural sobbing around the table was only interrupted by Jeff placing his finger over his trach, looking deep into my eyes as he spoke into the deepest places of my heart.

"I will always be with you, Honeybee."

The sea of emotions came crashing down in endless bursts of violent waves. The weight of his impending death overpowered us both. Every emotion, every beautiful memory, and every moment we would never share poured out of us. We didn't need to say it. We knew it would be the last birthday he would share with me.

I adored the depths of his unconditional and selflessly loving heart, which he expressed in countless ways to me daily. He made my birthday magical and unforgettable, even in the face of his impending death. The man I loved with every fiber of my soul tried to conceal the excruciating pain and exhaustion in each movement and word he spoke that day, but I sensed the suffering he tried to hide. I could see he wanted to take care of me that day, like he used to, and bring joy into our home one last time. I knew without a doubt that he pushed himself to his physical and mental limits to make my last birthday with him memorable.

The completed set of rings on my finger was not about a commitment; no two people could be more committed. Instead, the rings I still wear daily represent our journey of transforming our love from a fairytale into a battleground that weaved bravery and courage into our love story; those rings honor that love. Three years later, I still cherish that band as a reminder of how love can endure, flourish, and strengthen even when confronted with seemingly impossible challenges that nearly break you a thousand times over. They are a testament to our love that no distance or diagnosis could dictate our destiny or infect our love.

Journal

Some moments become etched in our hearts not because they are free of pain, but because they hold the purest expression of love in the middle of it. Reflect on a time when someone went beyond their own comfort or strength to show you how much you meant to them. How did that act shape the way you carry their love forward?

Chapter 19
FOUR WORDS

On April 14, 2017, Jeff asked, "Will you marry me?" in a picturesque lakefront location with Chicago's Magnificent Mile as our backdrop, and gray spring clouds floating across the Chicago skyline.

We were still living in two separate countries at the time, Jeff in Canada and me in Southern California. Jeff and our four children surprised me with the proposal while on a family vacation to Chicago. We had all flown in from opposite corners of North America for Easter weekend.

I was entirely in the dark about the life-changing event that was to transpire. He had hidden my engagement ring in Maddie's backpack to ensure I wouldn't accidentally come across it. All four kids had made matching signs on poster boards, rolled up and hidden inside their luggage. He had enlisted our kids to help make the weekend incredibly special.

Jeff was a hopeless romantic with whom I was hopelessly in love. He had packed hundreds of pictures of our life from the previous three years to bring on our trip. One night, he asked me to join him downstairs in the hotel lobby for a drink while the kids snuck into our room to create a wallpaper tapestry of our life woven together through pictures. They taped hundreds of photos throughout our room of our first few years together for me to cherish all weekend. I thought we had traveled to one of our favorite cities to visit my nieces, my brother Jeff's daughters, over a long Easter weekend. I was utterly oblivious to everything Jeff and the kids had secretly planned for me.

Before the trip, we'd hired a photographer to take family photos of me and Jeff and our blended brood of four. I didn't know that Jeff had secretly contacted the photographer to tell him to be prepared for a big surprise. Getting all six of us out of the hotel and ready on time was a bit of a struggle that day. We were slightly hungover after a late night partying with all the kids. But we eventually made it into our Uber, where we giggled, bickered, and sang to music as we gleefully bounced down Michigan Avenue toward Lakeshore Drive to meet the photographer.

We quickly piled out of the van one by one, like circus clowns exiting a car. The photographer immediately greeted us with a friendly smile; we were excited for a playful day by the lake, capturing more memories to hold in our hearts forever. Knowing the hidden purpose behind the photoshoot, our photographer set us up with our backs facing the city skyline so he could capture the joy of what was about to happen.

The breeze began to pick up in the windy city as thick, gray clouds threatened to sprinkle us with rain. We were running late, and nothing was going as we had envisioned for our planned family photo shoot. Even though everything was chaotic, our time together felt perfect. Jeff and I had always chosen to look at life through a unique lens; we looked at each frame as an opportunity to allow our story to magically unfold in a unique and unexpected way. We mapped things out but allowed flexibility to find its way in when an opportunity presented itself. Somehow, it always seemed precisely how God intended it; living by faith, not sight, served us well.

The photographer asked me and Jeff to set up first. He explained that he planned to take our photos before the kids joined in, and I thought nothing of it. Jeff gently held my hand, guiding me to a spot next to the water where the light spray of Lake Michigan playfully toyed with us as we stood on the concrete path. And then it happened.

Holding both my hands with all four children witnessing, Jeff began to speak softly to me, sharing how he loved our life. He told me he never knew his life could hold so much happiness—that I made every day worth living and that he truly came alive when he met me. Jeff was always so open with his emotions, able to reveal the deepest parts of his heart to me; he knew how to make my knees buckle and my heart skip a beat. As the photographer and kids looked on, that day was no different.

Jeff declared his devotion and undying love for me, then knelt on one knee.

"My Honeybee, I can't imagine another day without you in it. I don't want another sunset without you. I love you with everything I am. Will you marry me?"

My heart was bursting out of my chest as I began to cry, and I gushed out loud, "Yes. Absolutely, YES!"

All four children and everyone within earshot began to cheer, letting out screams of happiness, joining in our life-changing celebratory moment. Then, each of the children pulled out their poster boards with the words, "I said YES!"

That day, the rush of emotions that came with knowing we would spend the rest of our lives together felt like a dream; I was floating fifty feet above Michigan Avenue on a pillowy cloud all weekend. I was that obnoxious person, telling anyone who would listen to the glorious news of our beautiful engagement that I was the luckiest girl alive. I wanted the entire city to celebrate our love and the beautiful future that lay before us. That night, we all ate dinner at one of our favorite Italian restaurants in Chicago, La Scarola, and danced with the children and my nieces to live music, closing down the bars. We didn't want that day to end. Exactly one year and two weeks later, Jeff's cancer diagnosis flipped our world around and around like we were tumbling inside a washing machine.

"Today is the day."

I'd known these four words were inevitable as they sorrowfully crossed Jeff's lips.

My heart broke.

Four years, four months, and two weeks after Chicago, four powerful and profoundly different words forever changed my life. The four words Jeff spoke to me on September 1, 2021, through his tracheotomy, his voice weak and despondent as it crackled through the plastic hole in his throat, were in drastic contrast to his proposal and the emotions it evoked in Chicago.

I could barely comprehend his words and what was about to happen. I wanted to keep that terrifying information at bay and run as far as possible from it. I did not want to be the caregiver, advocate, or decision- maker anymore. I wanted to crawl into a dark hole and fall a million feet away from all my responsibilities.

We all wear many hats in life. My most valuable ones were mom, wife, friend, daughter, sister, aunt, niece, cousin, attorney, and business owner. But the hat I wore most often and with pride, those past few years, was caregiver and advocate. It's not a role anyone chooses; it chooses you. All my other hats had been hung up in the closet, collecting dust, patiently waiting for their turn to be put on again. But that day, Jeff asked me to put on a new hat I never wanted and prayed I would never have to wear.

How could I possibly find the courage to take off my hat as a wife, lover, caregiver, and best friend, to put on a hat that no one ever wants to wear … the hat of a widow? I wasn't ready. No one ever is. Seven and a half years together didn't seem nearly enough; we needed more time, and I needed more time. I didn't want to live a life without Jeff. He was my person, my everything. His energy breathed life into my lungs.

I rationalized that maybe it wouldn't exist or happen if I didn't tell anyone what he'd said, and I could somehow make it all disappear by ignoring it. There were times during those overwhelming years when I needed help because cancer and all it entailed were far too much, and I could feel myself crashing. During those times, when I could feel the pressure cooker building to its boiling point, I knew it was time to reach out for relief; family and friends always stepped up. My capacity was considerable, but it was not limitless. Over the years, I was never afraid to ask family or friends to step in and take over when my soul was depleted. But on our last day together, I couldn't pass the baton.

Part of me desperately wanted to give someone else that awful final charge. My mind wandered frantically, wondering if I could find the courage to go through with it.

How could I hand Jeff bottles to drink that would end his life? Would I carry an emotional burden for the rest of my life? Was it a burden, or was it a merciful gift? Was it the ultimate selfless act of love for Jeff?

I knew I couldn't allow someone else to step into my shoes. If I did, I recognized that it would be a decision I would regret for the rest of my life. I needed to find the courage to execute that one final act. I had taught my children that when making critical decisions, balance it out, weigh the burden versus the value, and look at the end goal. That day, I used the lesson I had taught my children as I considered the decision that lay before me. What was the burden and value of assisting Jeff to die with dignity?

I carried the weight of finding the strength to follow through on what Jeff and I discussed, and afterward, I would need to learn to move forward in life with no guilt or shame. I knew I needed to do that because the value in ending Jeff's suffering was immeasurable. There was no price too great for me to pay to end the torture his fragile and weakened body endured each day.

Looking forward months or years, if I had believed I would have had regrets, then my answer may have been different. I might not have been able to go through with it. That day, I had to search deep into my soul, find the unconditional love and strength that encapsulated our love story, and use that power for one last purpose: to end the unbearable suffering of the man who held my entire heart. In those minutes, I quickly and frantically balanced and rationalized the final act of our love story and whether I could find the courage to follow through.

I rapidly concluded that it was neither a burden nor a gift. Rather, it was my duty, honor, and final opportunity to show Jeff my absolute love and devotion. It would be our last act together.

We spent the past several months discussing Jeff's end-of-life choices, concluding that he wanted to live with dignity, not with pity or in the prison of constant pain that crippled him. The unbearable pain and deterioration of his body turned him into a walking shell of the man he once was, a virtual corpse that others felt sympathy for. Jeff was a prideful man and wanted his life to end with what dignity remained. The power he still held was to make that choice for himself.

To Jeff, living a life locked inside that prison with no ability to communicate or function was something he would not have accepted. That prison would be a life void of all dignity, pride, or value. It was non-negotiable.

Allowing him to become locked in that prison and to watch him live in that state only for my own personal gain of "hanging on" just a bit longer would have been selfish of me. And what exactly would I have been hanging onto? There were no more treatments, no surgeries, no hope. There was only pain; no joy, no quality of life. At times, he felt like an animal in a zoo, a spectacle for people to witness. Seeing his physical torture and mental anguish was cruel. There was only one way out of his painful prison.

Death.

I already experienced terminal cancer in 1995 when my brother was in a very similar state, but dying with dignity was not legal in California then. When my brother arrived home from the hospital to start hospice care, he became paralyzed from the waist down. He was not allowed to eat or drink, and he lay in a bed, suffering, just waiting to die. He would wander in and out of a lucid state, his body deprived of food and water. When he was barely conscious, he would awaken for a few moments, and I would speak to him. He gurgled through the fluid in his lungs—the sounds of groaning and immeasurable discomfort were his response.

Our conversations mostly involved reassuring him that I was there to comfort him so he wasn't alone. Inevitably, he would point to his mouth in a desperate plea for food or something to drink. He was only allowed ice chips out of concern for aspiration pneumonia, where one dies a painful death of suffocation when food or liquid is breathed into the lungs instead of being swallowed. I deceptively offered him a few ice chips for his thick, dry tongue to make him believe food and drink were being provided.

During his last several days, while he lay lifeless and in excruciating pain, he was thirsty and starving and continually reached for the morphine button to release more medicine. I knew there was a limit on his morphine release button; it only gave out a set dosage every so many minutes, but I would look into my brother's deep and desperate brown eyes that pleaded for mercy. Turning my head so that he couldn't see my tears, I pretended to push the button so he could try to fall asleep, believing relief was on its way.

I appeased his agony by telling him, "I just pushed it. More relief is coming soon," even when I knew relief was not coming until his last breath. This all felt inhumane.

Even thirty years after his passing, I can still see the desperation and misery in his eyes, pleading to make his suffering end. It took every ounce of my twenty-six-year-old self's courage to sit by his side daily, watching my best friend leave me between each long, labored breath, wondering which would be the last. There was no dignity, no mercy. It was our only option at the time. It felt remarkably cruel to allow a dying loved one to feel every ounce of breath stolen from his body as the torture of cancer painfully stole all his dignity and comfort with each tick of the clock.

Having been through such a horrific and heartbreaking end with my brother and now having Jeff tell me that today would be his last, I knew I could not succumb to that fragile inner voice of fear. I could not possibly condemn Jeff to an undignified and torturous end to an honorable life. We had choices, and his decision was clear. I needed to find the courage to honor his wishes bravely.

The illusory burden I was contemplating that I could carry into the future soon washed away, and a steady flow of compassion and love set in. Suddenly, I could see the value and power of having a choice. In the end, my brother became a victim of his cancer, and we all felt helpless. But this time, we were not powerless. It wasn't a burden; it was the last act of love I could grant to the man who had suffered, sacrificed, and fought with unimaginable heroism.

Jeff's powerful four words would forever drastically change everything. Those four words were the antithesis of the new beginning that the Chicago proposal had brought just four years prior. Acting upon them would freeze our love in time, and Jeff would forever remain four weeks shy of his fifty-third birthday. My horrible new beginning, without Jeff, was one I could barely breathe in; it suffocated me.

I began to hyperventilate as I allowed myself to really consider what that might look like. I would have to learn how to live a life alone without my love by my side every day. My mind began to go over every insignificant detail in our lives.

Did he show me where he kept the bulbs for the outside lights? How would I fix the fountain and pool equipment? Did he show me how he made the perfectly barbecued chicken or steaks that the kids and I loved so much?

I lamented how he took such care in everything he did for us. From fixing things around the house, to cooking the tastiest bacon, to making Canadian Caesars with the perfect splash of the bottled sauce we brought back from Grizzly Paw Pub in Canmore, where we'd spent many weekend getaways.

How could I figure out the recipe of love that he put into everything in our life together? I reflected.

Knowing Jeff's cancer was terminal for the past three and a half years, I thought I had asked all the questions and spoken all the last words, but I began to second-guess that. *What did I forget? Did I tell him today how much I loved and adored him and that I was so incredibly grateful for the life we'd created? Did I need to hear him tell me again how much he loved me?*

Deep down, I knew there were no more words we needed to say or hear. Thankfully, we shared the most intimate parts of our hearts every day through the years. But I could feel the seconds running away from me. Time was evaporating. I was grasping for air, for more memories, for more time.

Despite the many friends and family members who made up our solid circle of support, I was beginning to feel completely alone. I was about to start a new beginning I never wanted. There would be no more "Jeffanie," a fun term some friends referred to us by. No one would ever call me "Honeybee" again, and the other half of my heart would be forever still in time. I briefly admonished God for the first time in a very long time, realizing that the torture and agony of cancer had beaten us; we were genuinely defeated. There was no more fight, hope, or prayer to save him. He couldn't hold on any longer.

After running through everything in my mind, I finally made peace with those four horrible words. Today was the day Jeff let me know that his body could take no more suffering, and our valiant fight was over. We had overcome and heroically fought countless battles together. We'd defied so many odds over the past seven years. Today, no different than any other day, we would bravely carry out this last act together, lovingly holding each other until his last breath.

Today, we would lay down our swords and completely surrender.

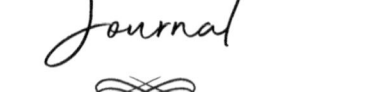

Some words change everything in an instant, sometimes bringing joy, sometimes breaking us open. Think about a moment when someone's words shifted the course of your life forever. How did you carry the weight or the gift of those words, and what did they teach you about love, courage, or letting go?

Chapter 20
TOODLE-OO

Jeff hated to say goodbye. Instead, he preferred to say "toodle-oo." From that very first day in the Las Vegas pool, he told me that sometime before his dad passed away, he began to avoid saying "goodbye." That word felt too final, so he adopted the lighthearted, optimistic send-off. He thought it somehow softened a painful goodbye. Everyone who knew Jeff knew toodle-oo was his personal touch of affectionately saying, "I'll see ya."

On August 28, I was driving home when I pulled up to a stoplight. A bright orange Jeep was waiting in front of me for the light to turn green; staring directly at me was a license plate that read "Tuduluh." I sat idling at the light, trembling. Clear as day, there was "my sign" to prepare. Sobbing uncontrollably, I looked up to the sky and asked God when it was going to happen. I knew at that moment that it was soon; Jeff's suffering was nearing its end.

When the light turned green, I captured a picture just before the car pulled away. I'm not sure why I took the photo—it just seemed like I needed proof of the sign I had just received. I told no one about the Jeep and the message on its plates until weeks after Jeff was gone. As I cried on that drive home, every fiber of my being knew that his last days with me were on the horizon.

The kids' summer breaks had ended, and they were returning to college. My knees buckled as they said their toodle-oo's to Jeff in the driveway. Witnessing the pain each one embodied, knowing they would never hug each other again, broke my heart; it was more than I could bear. I could feel my chest tighten, watching my children and Jeff hold each other. Their embrace was unlike before, neither wanting to be the first to let go. The hugs were filled with a longing for a future they would never see. The pain in their eyes was innocent and pure, unlike anything they had experienced. I wanted to protect them all from the heart-wrenching pain they were living, but I couldn't. It was yet another brutal part of cancer and Jeff's impending death. The beautiful love they shared made the pain unbearably intense.

On the morning of August 31, 2021, I received a stunning arrangement of pink and purple flowers that filled the house with a beautiful fragrance. The card read, "I love you so much, Honeybee. Love Always and Forever, Jeff." Later that day, Jeff made calls to the kids away at college. He made sure to spend time with each one, FaceTiming and sharing the pride and love that filled his heart. I sat in the room with him while he said his final goodbyes, telling each one how they had enriched his life and how blessed he was to have such incredible children to call him "Dad." They knew they would never hug their dad again, and Jeff knew he would never hold his children again. Every word and tear they shared shattered me.

Despite it all, I had somehow missed all the signs leading to the next day, September 1. I didn't see what was so apparent to me in hindsight. Maybe I was so blinded by fear and avoidance that I didn't allow myself to acknowledge the apparent indications of what was about to transpire. I couldn't sleep that night. Deep down, I must have known it was imminent, but still, I didn't connect the obvious dots. He was mapping it all out despite not having shared it with me. In hindsight, I can see he set a plan in motion days before he told me. Even in his final hours, Jeff made sure no detail was overlooked.

Unable to sleep that night, I looked at the clock. It was 12:22 a.m. I lay in bed holding my love's hands, as we did every night; my intuition must have known that our time together was slipping away. In the middle of the night, driven by instincts, I quietly reached for my phone. Something told me to snap pictures of our hands intertwined for one last sleep. I was subconsciously grasping to preserve our love, clutching at anything to hold onto and look back on.

When I awoke in the morning, I saw my love lying in bed so peacefully; it was an angelic state. His hands were in a prayer position resting on his chest, fingers intertwined as if he had awoken during the night and had begun to pray. My mind found tranquility in imagining that at some point in the evening, Jeff was praying to God for peace and strength for what the next day would bring.

When I saw him that morning, I wasn't sure if he had passed in the night because he was so still. Silently, I lay there breathless and terrified as I watched him lie peacefully still. Then I saw his chest move and realized with relief that he hadn't passed in the night. Many mornings had been filled with that frightening experience. Although I was relieved, I knew that meant another day of excruciating pain for Jeff. The conflicting emotions were ever-present. Once again, I reached for my phone and took a picture of him lying calmly, his hands still in a prayer position. Since then, I've read, "If you want to learn what someone fears losing, watch what they photograph." Those words were painfully apparent to my subconscious. I feared losing Jeff with every fiber of my being.

Later that morning, as I returned from my run, I would hear those four terrifying words cross Jeff's lips, leaving me frozen. My mind and heart could not comprehend what would soon transpire.

"Today is the day."

Those words hung in the air like an immovable black cloud. My heart raced, and tears poured down my cheeks uncontrollably. While Jeff held his composure, I could only imagine the heaviness of his emotions and thoughts. How much strength and heartache had it taken to contemplate and reach the decision to say those words at that moment?

It was time to open that brown bag I'd hidden so well. Jeff's mom and sister had been living in our home for a couple of weeks, like they had so many times over those years, supporting us in numerous ways. My friend, Michelle, was also with us most days that week, sitting downstairs quietly, working on her computer, and waiting to see if we needed assistance.

Michelle and I had been friends since our children were young. While I'm fortunate to have many close friends, our connection is unique. We met in 2006 when our children started Hebrew school, in kindergarten and second grade. Even though we were both raised Jewish, neither of us had the privilege of having our Bat Mitzvah as young girls. Michelle and I discovered that we both desired to have our B'nei Mitzvah as adults. In addition to achieving this personal milestone, we both felt it was important to set examples for our children while they were in the trenches studying themselves. After two years of rigorous studies, learning to read Hebrew, and finding a deeper connection with God, we had our B'nei Mitzvah together in 2010. Our daughters would have their B'nei Mitzvah in 2012, and my son in 2014.

Supporting each other in our forties to complete our dream as we led Shabbat services and read from the Torah, our bond deepened into a sisterhood. Over those fifteen years of friendship, we raised our children and stood by each other through divorces. Now, she walked resolutely beside me as I faced the most harrowing experience of my life.

Michelle called me days earlier and said she was coming over and would stay unnoticed in the corner of the family room, doing her work. If we needed anything, she would be there to assist us. Over the years, many friends and family members became caregivers for me, the caregiver.

When Jeff told me it was to be his last day on Earth, I panicked; I couldn't absorb the words he had spoken. I knew what he meant, but in denial, my heart was negotiating with my mind, grasping any possibility that what I had heard was a mistake.

Internally, I felt myself spinning out of control as I made every attempt to process the emotionally agonizing realization that we were living our last day together. I felt all the air in the room evaporate as I looked into my love's eyes and gasped for breath, firmly gripping onto our last seconds. There was no logical way to come to terms with what was about to take place; I had to propel myself to act and be "all in" in that moment, just like countless times throughout our relationship.

After frantically pleading with God to make it all disappear, I painfully forced myself out of a paralyzed state to be present with Jeff. Succumbing to my fears of what we were about to endure was not an option. He needed my loving strength one last time.

I gained my composure and then asked Jeff's mom and sister to join me upstairs so they could have their final cherished moments with him. While they were treasuring their last minutes, I made my way downstairs, where I found Michelle waiting and ready for whatever I needed. When I saw her, I collapsed and wept uncontrollably. I could barely breathe or walk on my own, and could feel my body give way. I struggled to see through my tears as she helped stabilize my body so I wouldn't fall.

Our home was calm, but my body was replete with chaos. Panic had set in. My mouth was dry as a desert and my throat began closing. I could feel my body wanting to shut down; I didn't want to face what was staring at me. At that moment, I wanted to run and escape that terrifying day, but I knew I couldn't give myself a choice. Giving myself a choice would have meant failing Jeff, and that was not an option; I couldn't let my love down.

There were no more choices, no more alternatives. I couldn't slow it down; it was the beginning of the end. I needed to find the strength to pull myself together so that in Jeff's final moments, he felt all my love and devotion surrounding him, just like in the past seven and a half years. I needed to focus on covering Jeff in my loving and protective arms, not my fear. I wished for Jeff's last moments on Earth to be filled with the knowledge that my love surrounded him for eternity. I wanted us to be in control of how our beautiful love story would end. That was important to Jeff, and I tried to find the strength to honor that.

My mind turned to the strength he possessed when deciding to choose a day. How does one decide to choose their last day on Earth? Very few words had been spoken about how we would select that fateful day. During the many weeks leading up to it, neither of us dared to discuss what his last day would look like or how he would choose it. It was too painful. Together, we had experienced so much love and agony over the years that I believed our hearts somehow knew with faith that the day would find us. That our hearts would guide us to the right day, just as they had guided us throughout our entire relationship.

Michelle and I entered the kitchen, and the adrenaline firing up deep inside me found its way to the surface, allowing me to concentrate on the unthinkable task ahead. By then, tears were pouring relentlessly down my face; I couldn't stop them if I tried. We went to the kitchen pantry, where I had carefully hidden that brown bag. It had been in our home for weeks, but I never broke the seal to look inside.

Trembling, I grabbed the brown bag off the shelf and set it on the kitchen island, where I collapsed, laying my face in my hands as I drowned in tears. I didn't dare open it; I couldn't stand to even look at it. Michelle stood silently beside me, giving me space and time to process what I had to do. It took several long and agonizing minutes, but finally, I forced myself to open the bag and read the instructions.

There were three small glass containers and a very specific set of instructions. As I read, my hands began shaking violently, and I couldn't make out the words; all the letters jumbled together. Tears blurred my vision, making it all the more difficult. Every bit of water poured out of me and onto the paper instructions, like a faucet I couldn't turn off. I tried desperately to read what I had avoided for so long, the instructions on how to end Jeff's suffering, but it was useless. I needed help. Jeff was waiting for me upstairs, and I knew I had to pull myself together.

I knew Jeff needed me, but at that moment, I couldn't find words. The weight of each movement was heavy and slow, as though I was trying to walk through quicksand. I was so thankful Michelle was there that day and quick to step in. She carefully took the paper out of my trembling fingers as I lost my composure and ability to function. She calmly and methodically read through everything, explaining that we needed apple juice to mix with the powdery concoctions in each small glass bottle. A specific timing was required between the three stages. As she explained each step and instruction, my ears heard every sound, but I couldn't process her words.

In hindsight, I should have opened that bag ahead of time and read the directions to be more prepared. But opening it was unimaginable until the day I was forced to. On my many runs in those final days, I prayed constantly that God would end Jeff's suffering. I did not want the responsibility of assisting the love of my life in dying. We had tried to avoid all of it for both our sakes.

The hospice team offered someone to assist us on the final day if we chose to go through with the process, but Jeff and I had declined. Although their assistance would have been helpful, we couldn't entertain the idea of a stranger in our home when we said our final "I love you." It is such a personal choice. We wanted to end our love story the way it started: deeply and madly in love, staring lovingly into each other's eyes, with our hearts pure and unfiltered. That was our beginning, and we would make it our end.

We talked very little about that day before it arrived, but one thing we knew for sure was that we wanted our last day together to be just like our first day. Just the two of us leaping together, having faith that our love would pave the way. We refused to let the fear of the unknown dictate our decisions.

We stood in the kitchen, Michelle reading the instructions, when I realized we had no apple juice to pour into each bottle. Michelle offered to run to the store up the road from my house and was soon out the door. Still in my sweaty running clothes from earlier, I wondered, *Is this the last vision of how Jeff will see me?*

My thoughts turned to what Jeff would see, feel, and hear in his final moments, his last breaths. I had never thought about those final hours; it was too painful. But at that moment, I only wanted to make it beautiful and meaningful for Jeff. Operating on nothing but adrenaline, I began to map everything out mentally and set the stage for his last hours. My mind turned to all the simple things Jeff and I loved.

Although it might seem vain, I didn't want to be sweaty from a run the last time Jeff saw me. While Michelle ran to the store for apple juice, I decided to take a quick shower. I was panicked and illogical, and nothing made sense. Precious seconds were slipping away, and my entire body began to freeze in shock for the second time that morning. An out-of-body experience took over as I walked into our bathroom. Taking off my running clothes while the water got hot, my mind wandered back in time through every special moment we had shared and our everyday life. Jeff was meticulous with every detail as he showered me with his love. He made the ordinary extraordinary and memorable, and I knew I needed to do the same for him in his last moments on this Earth.

I started considering the next few hours, his last few hours, and the last memories I would leave him with. We never discussed the details of his final day; we'd avoided everything about it. It was impossible for our minds to envision that day. From when we first met, all we did was fight for more time together, so to give in and accept the end had arrived was incomprehensible. Of all our difficult conversations over the years, discussing Jeff's last day was too heartbreaking for us.

My heart was on autopilot as I showered, leading me to what we loved most. Over the years, music allowed our minds to romanticize and hold each other close while opening our hearts to each other. Still running on adrenaline after exiting the shower, I instinctively grabbed my phone and created a new playlist. Intuitively, I titled it "Tuduluh." I added our favorite love, country, and spiritual songs that brought us peace. Keith Urban's "Making Memories of Us" came to mind first, reminding me of our first concert at the Calgary Stampede, then Luke Combs' "Better Together," followed by Lauren Daigle and MercyMe. The list grew long as I added more songs that had a special meaning to our life together and would allow love and peace to enter our hearts and the room.

Jeff loved playing that Keith Urban song to me repeatedly, singing each word as if it were his guide on how to love me. Each lyric in that song was our life. We had listened to it hundreds of times over the years. Jeff brought that song to life—the lyrics "loved me like no other," "winning my trust by making memories of us," and "I want to die in your arms" became a reality for us. Jeff made my world better than anything I had ever known. Being the hopeless romantics that we were, there wasn't a day we didn't expose our hearts to each other, which made our tragic ending so much more excruciating.

I was setting the stage just like Jeff would have done. Scanning the room, I wanted everything to be perfect. When you feel time frantically racing past you while trying to hold on with sheer desperation, you become another version of yourself that you don't recognize. I lost all control of my senses as my heart unraveled every beautiful memory we had created and all those that would be lost.

Navigating through unknown territory was terrifying. I wanted to control every second, yet I had lost all control. Isolation and fear crept deep inside of me, and I wanted to curl up in the fetal position in the corner of the room and wait for it all to be over. I felt paralyzed but knew I couldn't let the numbness take over. Instead, I became as reckless as a freight train. I forged forward, forcing myself to act so I wouldn't freeze up completely. My behavior wasn't logical, but neither was what we were about to do. That's when I turned off my emotions for a brief moment to accomplish a few last tasks for my love. Jeff sat in our bedroom chair, calmly watching me as I swirled around in chaos. The sense of peace that surrounded him slowly drew me in, as it had countless times before.

Initially, I'd been unable to calm down my racing heart as I became impulsive and crazed. I felt like I was watching myself from above, as if there were two of me in the room that day. The calm and loving version of me stood in the corner, allowing the panicked and hysterical version to grasp for air and time. The panicked me felt that I had to move; if I stopped, I was sure I would collapse.

I didn't think—I just acted. I ran downstairs and grabbed a candle, the portable speaker, and the flowers Jeff had sent me the day before. I carefully placed each item on a small table in front of Jeff to bring peace to the room. I put the beautiful bouquet next to the speaker and lit the blue, ocean-scented candle so that a calming, familiar smell filled the room. With serene, loving sounds and smells, we were ready for our closing act.

With the intimate scene perfectly set, I slowly closed the bedroom curtains. I got lost in the details for a few moments and numbly forgot the horror we faced. While I prepared the room, Jeff's sister and mom sat quietly with him and shared their last agonizing moments, saying their final goodbyes.

I heard Michelle downstairs as she returned from the store. Time felt like it was moving at lightning speed, yet simultaneously, the world around me was spinning in slow motion. It was like I was suddenly sinking into setting concrete and I couldn't escape. I was drowning. Today was the day, and now it was time.

I couldn't avoid the inevitable any longer. Death had caught up to us, and there was no more escaping. Words could not be found; we had no more time to buy. Writhing with anxiety and fear, I tried to slow my crying with long, deep breaths. I needed to be present for Jeff and myself. I was desperate to make sure every second we had left mattered. I couldn't fail him.

For weeks, the focus had been shifting from fighting for more time to processing and accepting that moment when we'd reached the end. Searching the depths of my soul, I prayed calmly, pleading with God for strength, courage, and peace so I could comfort Jeff in his final moments as he transitioned from this life into the next. He no longer needed to be brave. He could finally surrender, hand everything over, and breathe in his remarkable fifty-two years. Every internal conflict was reconciled, and his fight was over. His suffering would end today.

Michelle had already sent texts notifying family and friends that we were about to begin. Thinking of their pain from afar brought more heartbreak. Not being able to hold and comfort my children away at college while they were suffering was gut-wrenching. Jeff had spent the weeks prior telling those closest to him that he was choosing to die with dignity; there were no more options. It was vital for him that his loved ones knew and understood how hard he had fought and that he didn't want to leave them, but that the pain was unbearable, and with no quality of life remaining, he wanted his suffering to end. The loving support of all our family and friends had created a safe space for Jeff and I to follow through with such a heartbreaking decision.

In the kitchen, I placed all the necessary items on a bed tray to carry to our bedroom: the three small glass bottles of prescriptions, the apple juice, and the instructions. Each of the three steps needed to be administered precisely every thirty minutes. I was settling into what would transpire and was unsure of how I would monitor the time while absorbing every inch of Jeff and our last minutes together. Michelle offered to set a timer and ensured we had all the privacy we desired as she quietly sat in the back corner of our bedroom.

It was 4:21 p.m. when my body finally calmed, and the room felt right. I looked over at Jeff, who was watching me and allowing me to do what I needed so that I could find the peace to be in the moment with him lovingly.

It was then, with trembling hands, that I pushed play on the "Tuduluh" playlist. Keith Urban began to serenade us while, with hands shaking, I poured apple juice into the first glass container. The juice spilled everywhere as I tried to stabilize my unsteady hands. I looked into Jeff's eyes with a mixture of love and fear as I handed him that first drink, and Michelle set a timer. The first mixture was mild—a simple medication to help prevent nausea and vomiting.

Jeff and I cuddled into each other on the white chair, quietly looking into each other's dark browns and deep blues. As I lay beside my love, my heart couldn't take in what we had just started. My palms were slick with sweat, and my stomach was filled with knots of despair. I was engrossed with Jeff; nothing else existed but us and what little time was left.

We were in our bubble, completely lost in each other and tuning the world out, when Michelle's voice gently broke through.

"Steph, it's time."

I slowly peeled away from Jeff and stood. My body felt twice its weight. I sullenly walked over to the tray, tears streaming down my face, and poured juice into the second container. That second mixture was to slow down his heart and allow his body to fall into a peaceful state. When I turned back toward Jeff, I saw the same fear and despair I felt reflected in his eyes.

How do you soak in time when you're saying goodbye to the love of your life? Each set of thirty minutes felt crippling. As our love songs played, peace entered the room, and we held each other as our world slowly came to an end. Few words were spoken. We gazed into each other's eyes, our hands tightly intertwined as I draped myself over him. Our bodies became one as we listened to Luke Combs sing "Better Together."

The third and final bottle was the one that contained toxic medications that would end Jeff's life. The instructions were clear: Once he sipped the last bottle, there was no going back. The clock was racing past us, and soon, the second thirty-minute alarm came.

Michelle's voice was filled with compassion as she softly whispered, "Steph, it's time."

Dread filled my heart, and I could hear every beat sounding out the passage of our last minutes. I again peeled my body from Jeff's, and guttural sobs poured out of me while Jeff sat with a look of disbelief that he had reached his final thirty minutes. We were both in shock. With intense trepidation and trembling, I poured the juice into the final bottle. Tears streamed relentlessly down my cheeks as I turned back to Jeff, who sat frighteningly still, almost paralyzed. I could only imagine the extreme thoughts that he must have experienced.

Just before I gave Jeff the last drink, he removed his engagement ring and placed it on my finger. Removing his ring was another surreal moment I hadn't been prepared for, and it added more layers to my overwhelming heartache.

As though watching from outside my body, I saw my hand extend toward him as I handed the final bottle to Jeff. I felt absolute terror coursing through my body as he began to sip the deadly mixture while it bubbled from the toxic ingredients of the last vial.

Lying peacefully beside him, crying, I felt Jeff stiffen.

All at once, he shot up out of the chair, knocking over the flowers, the music, and the lit candle, startling everyone in the room. He'd had a burst of apprehension and panicked. We were too far into the process to stop and had only two choices: either I rushed him to the hospital or he finished the drink.

I held him, looked deep into his eyes, and said, "Honey, you don't have to do this, but we're too far along. We need to rush to the hospital or finish what we started. It's your decision; I will support your choice." He looked over to me for reassurance and wearily said, "Honeybee, what are we doing?"

Gazing into his eyes, I lovingly said, "Honey, you chose this path because of the excruciating and unbearable pain you're in every day. But if you want to stop, we must race to the hospital immediately."

A piece of my heart wanted to say, "Stop. Let's undo this and go to the hospital; I don't want you to leave me." But that would have been selfish of me, and in the end, it was not my decision. I had been suffering alongside Jeff for over three years, twenty-four hours a day, seven days a week. But it was his life and his choice. Once again, calm, he told me he wanted to complete what we had started. Hand in hand, we slowly walked back to the chair together. Michelle cleaned up the room, then walked out and closed the door behind her to give us privacy.

Jeff sat back down and finished drinking that last vial. I opened the bedroom curtains to allow the sunset to bring the last of the day's light into our room. Then I walked over and slid down next to Jeff into the overstuffed chair. We cuddled into each other, feeling the warmth of the bright summer sun shining upon us at that golden hour. I pressed play, and the song queued was "Peace Over You" by Here Be Lions. The words brought serenity into the room where Jeff and I lay together, tangled into each other. I could feel his body falling heavier onto mine as he fell into a serene state. The time between each breath he took began to lengthen. As each word of the song played, I could feel hope, joy, and peace enter the room as we held each other during Jeff's final minutes.

The room had transformed from fear, panic, and darkness into a calm, still, loving space. I watched his baby blues gaze into mine for the last time, our arms wrapped around each other with our fingers woven together, reminding each other that our love was always and forever.

Jeff looked at me lovingly, with both sorrow and peace. He tenderly spoke my name for the last time.

"I love you, Honeybee. There is no one in this world that I love more. I will love you always and forever. You are my Honeybee."

At 7:08 p.m., we breathed in our last sunset together as he fell peacefully asleep forever.

Jeff moved into God's loving grace and peace. His body suffered no more.

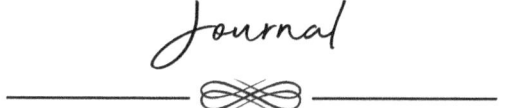

Sometimes, love asks us to be brave enough to say goodbye in a way that honors the life we've shared, even when it breaks us open. Think of a moment when you had to let go of a person, a season, or a chapter of your life, and write about how you found the strength to make that farewell as loving and intentional as possible.

Chapter 21

ASHES

Jeff's life had ended, yet I remained. The following day, the sun shone brightly through the bedroom windows; still, there wasn't enough light in the world to take away the icy darkness that consumed me. I'd been in a numb trance for hours, paralyzed and gazing despondently at the walls. My soul was filled with an endless abyss of hollowness without Jeff. The sounds of the world around me seemed muffled, and the room felt cold and lifeless. The all-consuming silence surrounding me that morning would become a part of my daily routine, my new normal.

My eyes and mind began to find daylight, just as a horribly vivid memory washed over me from the night before. Walking next to the gurney that wheeled Jeff out our front door and over the welcome mat, I kissed his cold lips gently for the last time.

In the morning light, I shivered and reached for Jeff's phone. I found it lying on top of the flat, untouched sheets. His phone felt like an extension of him, like I had a piece of him lying beside me in bed. My body and heart were in shock, realizing I would never open my eyes and see signs of my love throughout our bedroom and home. I wrapped my arms gently around his pillow, breathed in, and committed every scent to memory while I lay in silence. There were no more tears, just a deep numbness consuming my entire body. Lying in the fetal position before dawn, aimlessly gazing at the ceiling, I was in a state of shock and disbelief. I desperately yearned to hear, "Good morning, Honeybee!" followed by a soft kiss. But I never would again, and the thought was crushing.

No more good morning kisses with Jeff wrapping his long arms and legs around me while we cuddled into each other. Nothing was more important to Jeff than ensuring time stood still when we were together. Unlike the night before, when I frantically wanted time to stop so I could hold onto him for eternity, I had abruptly become desperate for time to race by. I wanted to find a way to make the shocking pain that coursed through my body disappear. My heart had been shattered into a thousand tiny pieces, and I struggled to find my way past the heavy weight of suffocating loss.

Three and a half years earlier, my grieving began when Jeff received his terminal diagnosis. Denial, anger, bargaining, depression, and acceptance were emotions that Jeff and I lived with daily. Even though it demolished our hearts and our world, we learned to create beauty amidst our heartbreak and grief. Despite the battles we faced during those challenging years, the gratitude I found would prove vital in my healing, but the process would be slow.

After his death, life initially felt pointless. There seemed to be no value in my days, no more purpose. Throughout the three and a half years leading up to Jeff's death, I had time to prepare for that moment when my life would start over without him, but I realized after he was gone that no amount of time would have been enough to say goodbye and let him go. He was my life and my future, and he held my entire heart.

The morning after Jeff passed, and in the days that followed, people called and walked in and out of our home ceaselessly. Oddly, I don't recall many of those initial days. I began living unconsciously in each moment as the hours passed, without much concern for the outside world. I interacted and spoke with those present, but my mind was entirely absent. With my kids away at college and no more advocating or caregiving to keep Jeff alive, I felt I had no purpose moving forward. The strength to retrieve and replenish my depleted soul had suddenly vanished.

Having experienced many losses, I knew that for me, there was only one way to truly find my way out of that dark pit of heavy and painful sorrow. I couldn't ignore the pain or pretend it didn't exist; I needed to address it head-on. But that first morning and for the next many days, I needed to allow myself space and grace to do whatever was necessary to breathe and survive while my heart suffered. Every heavy thought came at me in slow motion, and the most ordinary routines—even pulling the sheets back to get out of bed—felt like an overwhelming challenge.

My oldest childhood friend, Margo, was in my home within hours of me waking up that first morning. She lifted me in my darkest hour. Time was distorted, and everything felt excruciatingly slow. I was paralyzed with fear of my new life without Jeff but grateful to have my dear friend by my side. I was desperate to leave our home where every beautiful memory tore at my heart, so Margo's presence was a huge relief. Opposing emotions consumed me in those early days, and she stayed close, walking with me through much of it.

One of my first agonizing responsibilities was to make arrangements for Jeff's cremation. I dreaded the thought but was determined to complete the devastating task hastily. Margo helped me with the details, and together, we found a beautiful set of urns online: a large one for my home and a small, purse-sized one that I could carry with me. After we finished that heart-wrenching job, I needed to get out of the house; there was a sense of the walls closing in on me.

Driving Jeff's truck brought comfort and a feeling of closeness to him, so I grabbed his keys and a couple of his Kokanee (Canadian beers) and drove us to his favorite beach in Laguna. We sat on the beach drinking Kokanee and watching the waves crash down. The smell of the salty ocean, as it surged in rhythmic movements, flooded my soul with memories of Jeff. I allowed myself to do whatever felt right at that moment to get through the pain. I played in the sand like a child and did everything my soul needed to survive that day.

Knowing my children were also suffering from afar, I wanted to be with them to support them in their sorrow. I recalled what it was like to lose my brother while I was in law school; I knew they needed comfort. Within days of losing Jeff, I decided to visit each of them at college and quickly booked flights for the end of September. First, I flew to see Maddie in Idaho, where she was four weeks into her first semester of grad school at Boise State University. Then, I flew to Nashville to be with Jake, who had transferred to Vanderbilt University his junior year. It was October 1—Jake's birthday and Parents Weekend; I was grateful to be with him for both occasions.

Spending a week with each of my kids was a great source of healing for us all. We cuddled through the tears, recalling stories as we fondly remembered the man who had profoundly touched our souls. During that time, I was preparing the details for Jeff's memorial services, which we called "celebrations of love," in Canada and California, and Maddie and Jake each expressed their desire to honor Jeff at both services by sharing how he'd positively impacted their lives.

Jeff passed on September 1, and for the next three months, I continued to power through nonstop while making all the arrangements and planning both services. After flying home from visiting Maddie and Jake, I finished the arrangements for Jeff's first service in Canada on October 15 and the service in California on November 5.

After a devastating loss, many painful yet inevitable firsts are marked in our minds, such as birthdays, anniversaries, and holidays. Those are the ones we anticipate, and I found there was no easy way to move through them except to get in the muddy trenches and work through each one. But the things that most crippled me were the unexpected firsts.

Several weeks after Jeff was gone, I finally felt it was time to remove all the pills and medical supplies from our home. I became anxious to complete the devastating task. Living with daily reminders of the torturous pain his body endured was not comforting or healing. My cousins Vanessa and Rudy patiently spent days helping me box up and dispose of every reminder of cancer, from the medical supplies to the dozens of pill bottles. I knew they were unnecessary and would only hinder my healing; each item dredged up memories of Jeff's suffering. Within a couple of months, we had removed them all.

Another unexpected first occurred a few weeks after Jeff had passed when I went to the pharmacy to pick up a prescription. Walking toward the counter, I became overwhelmed with emotion when I saw the pharmacist who had memorized our names and Jeff's date of birth. Jeff was his regular patient. Having seen him multiple times a week for years, he had become a friendly, familiar face. Approaching him that day, I began to sob uncontrollably in the middle of the store. He lowered his eyes as he read the news in my reaction. He quickly walked over and gave me a warm hug.

I had been completely taken aback by grief that day. Sitting in my car after getting my prescription, tears continued to flow, and I wondered how many more surprise reactions I would find myself having in the future. It wouldn't be long before I was once again blindsided by grief.

The next time, it occurred on my trip to Canada for Jeff's service. I had prepared myself for being in his hometown, knowing Jeff wouldn't be at the airport waiting to hold me like so many times before. I felt confident and strong when the plane touched down that afternoon, but when I exited the plane, an unexpected rush of emotions diminished me to a fragile state. I had just walked past the exact spot where, seven years earlier, Jeff had embraced me on my first trip to Canada. That day, we'd danced at the airport while a country band played songs welcoming visitors to town for the Calgary Stampede.

My knees went weak, and my whole body began to shake. Fighting back tears, I forced my way through the crowd of passengers and found a private corner. There, gasping for air, I bent down into a ball, engulfed by a wave of panic. Memories of Jeff flooded over me, and I wept bitterly. The crushing pain I felt that day had become an integral part of my healing process in learning how to survive without him.

Following the services in Canada and California, I stared down the dark tunnel leading into my first holiday season without Jeff. Those first holidays were excruciating, from hearing music to seeing decorations in the stores and all the holiday lights hung cheerfully from rooftops. January 1 couldn't come fast enough. With the end of 2021 approaching and the kids and I wanting to escape the sharp void of Jeff's presence, we decided to explore Sun Valley, Idaho.

Nothing could alleviate the torturous pain I felt, but getting out of town and escaping the memories in our home was a welcome distraction. The unfamiliar scenery brought some relief and levity, making Jeff's absence less obvious. It was challenging navigating my grief while simultaneously supporting my children's pain; I wanted to selfishly abandon all my parental responsibilities and crawl into a hole. I forced myself out of my self-pity and back into the role of mom; we found a balance during that delicate and complicated time.

I found the security I needed in surrounding myself with people who allowed me to do or say anything I needed while finding my way through that nightmarish time. I never had to weigh my thoughts, actions, or words with friends and family. They were a great source of comfort while I navigated through unknown territory. They allowed me to work through the insecurities and uncertainties of a new version of myself, which emerged over the next year.

After the holidays, I was home in California and back to my regular life. With the new year beginning, I began to find my way out of the heavy, dark cloud that followed me. It had been four months since Jeff passed away. I was slowly recovering and healing from the massive loss when I decided it was time to return to routines I knew would help restore joy and hope to my soul. Regardless of how many years passed, I would always carry the grief with me as a badge of love and honor. But getting stuck in grief is not a part of my DNA. Nothing felt the same, and nothing was normal anymore. My love was gone forever, and the gaping hole felt endless. I knew I had to push myself and start finding purpose once more. Pockets of joy would be mine again one day, but I needed to force myself to keep moving forward and find something else to focus on rather than the excruciating hole in my heart.

Turning to one of my reliable lifelines, I leaned into running. My thirty-one-year-old niece, Samantha, asked if I would train with her for a half-marathon. It would motivate her to get back on the road and provide me with a good distraction from the heavy grief I was living with each day. It was just what I needed. We planned to meet for an April race in Key Biscayne, Florida. It would be our second time running a half-marathon together; the first was in Myrtle Beach, South Carolina, seven years earlier. Meeting my niece at a fun location was a great way to combine one of our passions and give us quality time together.

Over the years, I had run over a dozen half-marathons and two Ragnar Relay races. I had taken up running in my early forties; before that, I never ran. I would even say I despised running; nothing about it appealed to me. But now, I loved running. It tested my perseverance, especially starting later in life. When I first attempted to run, I could barely go three blocks without stopping. Being an athlete my entire life, I was surprised at the higher level of endurance, mental toughness, and strength that running required from my body compared to other sports. Initially, I found it so difficult that I almost gave it up several times. But after keeping with it for weeks, I began to get the runner's highs that I had heard about. That was it—I was hooked. I continually stacked on more blocks and miles until I ran my first half marathon at forty-four.

Throughout Jeff's illness, running became an instrument that brought me solace and peace to support him through our battle. Running allowed me to replenish my soul and come home whole and ready for the challenges we faced. Now that he was gone, I believed that running would help replenish my soul once more, helping to ease some of my grief and pain.

With the new year beginning, I regularly sat in my grief alone, barely going through basic daily activities. Some days, I went into our business, which provided a much-needed distraction, but other days, I felt accomplished simply showering and brushing my teeth. I felt it was time to get myself out of that unwanted space of hopelessness; I needed to find my purpose again. My inner strength had given way to isolation and despair, and I needed to recoup it. I knew running was just the thing, and preparing for a race with my niece was the perfect motivation.

The most memorable race happened during my first visit to see Jeff in Canada. The Calgary Stampede half-marathon had been a joyous occasion as I ran with him cheering me on. It was early in our relationship, and we were learning each other's funny little quirks and patterns. On the morning of the race, we were enjoying each other's company and lost track of time. We were left to frantically "race" to the race when we realized how late it was. Upon arrival, Jeff wheeled the truck up as close as he could get me, ran over a few curbs, opened the door, and said, "Run." I thought to myself, *Duh, that's what I'm here to do.* I looked back at him with a grin of annoyance. "Seriously, babe, this is how I'm going to start my first trip to Canada?" Leaning on the steering wheel, he tilted toward me, almost pushing me out, and said, "Yep, get out of the truck and getter done. Run, Honeybee." I ran from the truck to the start line, barely arriving before they closed it off.

Running that day, I laughed at how annoyed and in love I was with Jeff. He somehow found me at every possible point on the beautiful trails of Calgary and cheered me on like it was the Olympics; he was remarkably endearing. After the race, we found an excellent place for a bison burger and beer in the heart of downtown Calgary, surrounded by a litany of Stampede festivities, haystacks, and cowboys.

The Calgary Stampede is the world's largest outdoor rodeo, spread over ten days. It was unlike anything I had ever experienced; the entire area had been transformed into an urban rodeo with concerts and cowboy gear spread throughout the city. When I arrived at the airport in Calgary, I walked through the doors and was greeted by a live band welcoming the passengers from our plane. As I looked for Jeff in the sea of people, I was lassoed by a couple of cowboys while a band played in the background. Jeff immediately pulled me from the rope and started dancing with me to the sound of a fiddle while someone put a cowboy hat on my head.

Reaching back to those memories, I tried to find the joy I had felt during that half-marathon in Calgary. But this time, I was without Jeff. Running was the one thing that always seemed to draw the pain from my soul and refill my cup. Everything about the idea of training for a race with my niece felt apropos. We decided to turn our new journey into a girls' trip. Samantha's mom, my good friend Stephanie, would join us to cheer us on as we ran. The plans and my training began with the new year.

I reminded myself how to train for a race, bought two new sets of running shoes, and created a running schedule. Runs were like personal therapy sessions filled with tears and smiles. During each mile, I processed the loss of Jeff, the memories we had created, and what my future looked like without him.

Throughout my runs, peaceful thoughts and recollections of the beautiful life we'd shared sank in, and I was reminded of our trip to Boston. One day, while on a training run, an idea hit me like a ton of bricks: I could turn the race in Florida into a fundraiser to honor Jeff and give the proceeds to the Cam Neely House Foundation. That way, our donation could assist other families battling cancer and facing the same challenges we did.

The months of preparing turned into a pivotal point of healing for me as I put in 225 miles of training, which gave me endless hours alone on the pavement, meditating on my memories of Jeff. With the support of two women I adore and a multitude of family and friends lifting me up, the race became a powerful and paramount event in my recovery. During the three months of training, Samantha and I checked in on each other regularly. She battled the bitterly cold New York winter, and I, on the other hand, found relief in the California sunshine. Time passed quickly, and soon, I found myself leaving for Florida.

Key Biscayne is a picturesque place for an adventure, with miles of white sand to walk along and cool ocean breezes that sweep in to bring relief from the hot sun. Over the marathon weekend, the three of us shared intimate conversations and healing laughter over meals and wine. We sprinkled in walks along the warm beaches, leaving our footprints under each wave. It was a time that rejuvenated my spirit and brought joy into my life again.

When the race day arrived, I woke up well before sunrise and sat alone on the hotel balcony. With thoughts of Jeff, I listened to the ocean waves crashing in the early morning hours and fought back tears. He would've loved it there. Watching the sun slowly lift on the ocean's horizon, I shared with him how badly I wanted him on the route that day, cheering me on once more. I knew nothing would ever be the same. That morning, I put on my running pants, which I had bought for that race in a bright blue color that Jeff loved. I attached my running bib and neatly tucked a small pouch of Jeff's ashes into my pocket. I carried him with me during the race and could feel his presence, giving me strength throughout each of the 13.1 miles.

From start to finish, Samantha and I ran side by side, encouraging each other. Sharing that time was invaluable. After the race, I walked with Samantha and Stephanie along the white sand and popped a bottle of champagne. We took turns drinking from the bottle of bubbly, toasting to each other and Jeff. During that walk, I realized I had turned my pain into purpose, running in Jeff's honor and raising funds for the Cam Neely Foundation.

I couldn't fully know what would evolve when that journey began months earlier. During my training leading up to the race, perseverance broke through the pain on those miles of reflection, releasing the tension from my shoulders. The guttural sobbing I'd experienced on my first few training runs subsided into soft, flowing tears intermittently. My every waking moment was no longer concentrated on the devastating pain and sorrow I had been carrying for the past four years. I no longer focused on myself and Jeff alone, but instead shifted my thoughts to others and how I could help them through my pain.

While training, I came up with the idea of doing something unique that would push me far outside my comfort zone. After the race in Key Biscayne, Samantha and Stephanie flew back home to New York, and I caught a flight from Miami to the island of Antigua for my first solo vacation. There, I would continue my healing.

The thought of taking a trip alone brought conflicting emotions; I was terrified of going to an island alone, but I was exhilarated by the unknown possibilities. The idea of doing whatever I wanted whenever I wanted felt like the perfect antidote for my ailing heart and depleted soul. Landing alone on an island where no one knew my story or my pain, and I could share as little or as much as I chose, was appealing.

I got off the plane in Antigua and walked to a cab. The warm island breeze invigorated my soul, and my inner peace began to emerge. It was much like the trip to Las Vegas when I met Jeff; I desperately yearned to rediscover my youthful and playful old self.

I met groups of women friends at the pool and beach that week in Antigua. I accepted a few invitations to dinners, hikes, and excursions. I met a woman at the resort when I asked her to assist me with putting sunscreen on my back. She was visiting the island with her husband, young adult children, and some family friends. After enjoying a long conversation, we got to know each other a bit, and she invited me to join their group for dinner and music at sunset on the other side of the island at Shirley Heights.

Shirley Heights is a restored military lookout that's been turned into a popular restaurant and bar where tourists and locals gather. Perched high on a hill facing west, its breathtaking panoramic views of the harbor, rolling hills, and magnificent sunsets make it the perfect spot to enjoy an evening on the island. Throughout the night, the smell of barbecue jerk chicken and ribs wafted in the air, and colorful tropical drinks flowed while Caribbean music infused the night with vibrant rhythms. We danced and laughed the night away, watching the sun disappear like a fireball melting into the sea. The new friends I made that week invigorated my soul with laughter and the fresh vibrancy of friendship.

Spontaneously throughout the week, I became more energized and alive, with each impulsive decision revitalizing me to my core. Freely hopping on a catamaran, I snorkeled around the island in the crystal-clear turquoise waters, took long walks on the pristine white beaches, and engaged in lighthearted conversations while sipping prosecco. It was precisely what I needed to reignite my spirit. On my last morning in Antigua, while enjoying the warmth of the morning breeze and the Caribbean sun, I suddenly remembered that a trip to the Caribbean had been an unchecked item on Jeff's bucket list.

I had taken Jeff's small, pocket-sized urn in my purse to comfort me as I traveled. Before leaving for the airport, I asked one of my new friends if she would join me on the beach and videotape while I honored Jeff. With the salty sea water spraying in the warm morning sun and tears flowing gently down my cheeks, I left a tiny part of Jeff in the Caribbean.

That trip would be the first of many I would check off Jeff's bucket list in his honor. Taking time alone in reflection and the freedom that came with it touched my soul deeply. It was not only cathartic but also liberating as I discovered a new version of myself. I didn't know what I was looking for or what I might find on that solo trip, but it nourished my soul and liberated me from the prison of sorrow and despair I'd been living in.

By then, I was coming up on my first birthday without Jeff, so I planned a trip to Chicago with my children. The idea snuck up on me while we were there to find the exact place where Jeff got down on one knee five years earlier. Together, the kids and I found the spot. There, on the edge of Lake Michigan, looking back at the city skyline, my heart began to pound out of my chest. I found the small urn in my purse and decided it was a perfect place to leave some of Jeff's ashes.

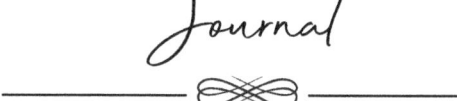

Grief can feel like an anchor that keeps us in place, but sometimes small acts of love, like honoring a memory or carrying someone's spirit into a new experience, can start to lighten the weight. Think about a way you've carried a loved one forward with you, whether through a tradition, a symbolic gesture, or an adventure, and write about how it helped you feel connected while moving ahead.

Chapter 22
A SECOND SUNRISE

That first year was ending, and the raw, intense sorrow had slowly transformed into hope and joyful new memories. I had no expectations of what the first year or the rest of my life would look and feel like, but I was surprised to find myself enjoying moments of true happiness again. It was still crushing to know Jeff would not be a part of my life moving forward, but I was optimistic for the future.

I allowed myself to work through each emotion and feeling. Mapping and planning things out took a back seat to improvisation while I reinvented myself without Jeff. People often asked me if I planned to move and sell my home or business, but I was in no hurry. I would know if and when the time was right. Oddly, I found comfort in not knowing what was around the corner and whether I would choose to embrace it or not. Although I sought advice from those closest to me, it was liberating and terrifying to know that I alone could make every decision on how my future unfolded.

After making it through that first painful year, I was happy with my life and how it was moving forward as I discovered joy in the new version of myself. I was creating new routines, allowing happiness and laughter back into each day, taking solo trips, and spending time with family and friends. What I'd had with Jeff was a powerful love, one that I wish everyone could experience. Before he passed away, I knew that I had no desire ever to date again; I had lived what others may call a dream. Putting my heart at risk felt unnecessary. I was recovering, and I was happy. That was enough.

I don't recall precisely when, but something changed unexpectedly toward the end of that first year. It was as if a light switch abruptly flipped inside my heart. Maybe it was the hopeless romantic in me or the yearning for that inexplicable feeling of exposing my heart and being vulnerable and safe with another person. Whatever it was, I felt ready to seek love once more. Initially, I was taken aback by this new desire. I weighed the risk to my heart against the reward of finding love again. Being a person in love with love, I suppose I shouldn't have been so surprised by my willingness to put my heart on the line.

The fear of opening my heart and facing the potential pain of losing someone I love again far surpassed the anxiety of stepping back into the dating world. When I considered dating, overwhelming thoughts swirled through my mind. *What if something were to happen to him, and I would have to experience all the heartbreak and pain again? Was I ready for that?*

I spent weeks considering the idea of dating again and all the possibilities that came with it, both positive and negative. I concluded that if I found another love to share my life with, the reward of being in love would outweigh the potential pain of another loss. I couldn't let fear fuel my decisions, so I threw caution to the wind and took the guard off my heart.

After gaining clarity, I called my children and shared with them that I was ready to date. I wasn't looking for anyone's permission, but I wanted their blessing—a reassurance that they were prepared for me to explore finding love again. I knew their hearts were still healing alongside mine, and I needed to know they were emotionally ready to accept this in their lives, too. I needed their support to enjoy the process of seeking a partner with whom I could share the second half of my life.

After giving me their blessing, they made a simple suggestion: I move my rings to my right hand since I was not looking for a man who wanted to date a married woman. I knew that I would never take off the rings Jeff gave me to honor our love. To this day, I still wear those rings proudly on my right hand. As I spoke to them about dating, I was surprised and overjoyed by their support. We laughed together as my children, now in their twenties, shared their dating advice.

I married my ex-husband in the nineties, and hadn't dated in thirty years. Following my divorce, I met Jeff by happenstance while in Las Vegas. Privately, I hoped I would get lucky twice with another chance encounter. However, not being one to wait for things to happen, I jumped headfirst into the new and intimidating world of dating apps. Knowing a few couples who had met online, I felt optimistic. So, one evening, while home alone, I opened a bottle of wine and Match.com. With a glass of liquid courage in hand, I apprehensively created a dating profile.

It was honest, straightforward, and playful. I knew what I wanted in a committed partner and wasn't afraid to ask for it. I was filled with so many mixed emotions: excited at the possibility of finding love again, yet petrified that I could lose a person I love once more. I compartmentalized and pushed my fears aside to enjoy the new dating experience with a lighthearted approach.

While online dating, I was reluctant to give my number to anyone until I had fully deposed them. Cautiously and slowly, I shared personal information as I got to know each person through phone calls and texting. Despite knowing that I could block anyone at any time, I still felt that giving out my number was like inviting them into my home. A few times, I was forced to block men's numbers.

Some men I interacted with were not on the same page as me; they were either not serious about finding a dedicated life partner, or I sensed they had something to hide. I took a pass if they were uncomfortable answering reasonable questions or if my intuition told me they were not being forthright. If I was going to expose my heart to someone, I believed there was no question off limits. Although I had heard some success stories, I'd also heard dating nightmares, so I always put my safety first. I researched as much as possible, using Google and social media to verify their information. I drove myself to each first date and gave my girlfriends the individual's information and our location in case of an emergency.

I went on a handful of first dates and found it unnerving and exhilarating. When I went on my very first date, I was extremely nervous. My heart raced while I got ready and fretted about what to wear, ensuring my hair and makeup were on point. When I arrived at the restaurant, my worries changed from myself to the man I was meeting. Suddenly, I wondered, Would he look like his pictures and match his profile? *Would I find that intangible connected feeling I desired?*

I arrived early at the charming restaurant he'd chosen in Laguna Beach and ordered a lemon drop martini at the bar to calm my nerves. When my date arrived, I was pleasantly surprised to find that he looked just like his profile: tall, attractive, and tastefully dressed. That evening, immersed in great food, wine, and engaging conversation, my nerves quickly faded. We sat at a quiet table for hours, and when the restaurant closed, he offered to walk me to my car.

Leaving the restaurant that night, I was proud of myself for choosing a great person to have a first date with. We strolled through the parking lot, his arm gently guiding me, as I felt that first date buzz. It was something I hadn't felt in years, and the energy building deep inside was electrifying. When we arrived at my car, he thanked me for a great time and leaned in for a kiss. Afterward, he hugged me tightly. With his strong arms around me, I felt safe. I stepped back in an effort to pull out of the hug, and his entire body suddenly went limp. He was heavy and fell onto me, knocking me backward as he passed out in the middle of the parking lot.

I stood there stunned for a moment. Initially, I thought it was a joke, but when I called his name, there was no response. Uncertain of what was happening, I began to panic; my mind violently jolted back to all the emergencies I'd experienced with Jeff. Dread washed over me. Had this man just had a heart attack or stroke? My fears peaked, and I grabbed my phone to call for help when he came to. Embarrassed, he said it had never happened before but refused to let me call 9-1-1. I helped him, offering him water from my car and a ride home. He declined my offer to drive him home, insisting he was fine. We never had a second date, but that night will always stay with me; the ending is something I will never forget.

As I continued dating online, I learned that being a widow posed additional concerns. I quickly realized that some men on the site would try to take advantage of me, assuming I was more vulnerable and an easy target. There was also the issue of people judging me, similar to when I divorced after a twenty-one-year marriage and started dating Jeff. While navigating the uncharted territory of self-discovery after losing Jeff, I dealt with others wondering how I could date again after having such an all-consuming love with him. Several people inserted themselves when I began online dating, thinking they had a say in how I lived my life and decided what my happiness looked like. During those pivotal times, some questioned my decisions and audaciously injected themselves into my shoes. I quickly realized that their misplaced judgment was not my concern. I didn't need to explain myself to anyone, and I didn't need their approval. My only concern was my happiness and that of my children.

On my new dating adventure, I found myself having fun. I met some nice men, but no one seemed a fit until I met Tim. We texted on the app for weeks before I felt comfortable enough to give him my number. We later joked that I was like Fort Knox, holding onto my privacy. It wasn't until months later that he shared he'd only stayed on the app to get my phone number. Once I gave him my number, he closed his dating account. Tim had been looking for someone for a while and was tired of the dating apps; he felt he was done if it didn't work out for us. From the start, I found his confidence and certainty in what we had extremely attractive. He knew what he wanted and was willing to immediately commit his efforts to what we started.

After I gave him my number, we talked on the phone and set our first date. We met at an outdoor patio in Orange County on a sunny afternoon for a glass of wine. His meticulously styled, light, wavy brown hair, his warm hazel eyes, and his fit body matched his profile; he was clearly an outdoor and fitness enthusiast like me. His shoulder and bicep muscles bulged from his fitted black t-shirt, neatly tucked into his khaki green shorts. He had a polished yet casual appearance and a joyful, calming demeanor that instantly drew me in. I walked up to him smiling, and his face broke into a wide, genuinely kind grin. He gave me a welcoming hug radiating affection, instantly putting me at ease.

We sat on the patio talking for hours, discovering more about each other and sharing a few funny dating stories. Tim, once married, had been single for over a dozen years. He'd dated occasionally but never found someone special to settle down with. Everything about our first date seemed right; I felt a peaceful sense of security with Tim. After our first date, I walked away feeling a genuine connection. It was invigorating.

Tim was a true gentleman. It wasn't until our third date that he leaned in to kiss me; he wanted to take things slow, not wanting to scare me off and ruin the possibility of a future. On the phone one evening, a month after we started dating, Tim told me about a planned work trip to Marrakech, Morocco. The trip was only weeks away, and he wanted me to join him. In the back of my mind, I wondered how many others he had asked over the years to join him on work trips. I didn't want to be another notch in someone's belt. I also didn't want to get stuck across the world with some guy I barely knew.

I wasn't dating for a free meal or an exciting trip. I was looking for substance in a sincere, loving relationship that was authentic. The idea of traveling the world together after only having known him for a few weeks was terrifying and exhilarating. Although I felt safe with Tim, I thoroughly checked his background after hearing dating horror stories. Tim's background and everything he shared with me checked out, so after several more dates and hours of conversation, I threw caution to the wind and accepted the invitation. I didn't know he had already added my name to the travel guest list before the window to bring a plus-one closed.

We excitedly packed and planned our two-week adventure. I held my breath at times as excitement and nerves overwhelmed me. I knew

I couldn't let fear or anxiety hinder the unique opportunity to find love. Together barely two months, we eagerly mapped out our trip across the world, booking flights and hotels as we added on Portugal before Morocco, researching adventures in enchanting castles and romantic coastlines.

The trip was a wonderful and exhilarating way to grow our relationship. We learned many things about each other in such a short amount of time as we traveled the world. We climbed fortresses and castles in Lisbon, took in the breathtaking landscape of the Algarve Coast, and went tandem kayaking through the Benagil caves and the São Rafael grottos, with illuminating water guiding our path. We navigated the intimidating and rocky ocean waters, ducking underneath sharp edges while exploring caves. Tim stayed close by my side, confidently reassuring me and calming my nerves when we got close to the rocky edges.

We found secluded beaches to soak in the sun and waves. In those private moments, I remember looking around me and at Tim, then wondering at God's graciousness in bringing someone so good into my life once more. My gratitude was overflowing at the realization that I had been blessed twice.

Exploring the world together, we opened our hearts and learned about each other's unique approaches to life. With each day that passed, our love grew. Not every adventure was lighthearted and fun; we also learned how we handled stressful situations differently.

While in Portugal, Tim was driving our rental car one afternoon when he pulled to the side of the road to look up a dinner destination on his phone. He hadn't noticed a gaping hole directly in front of us, hidden by the car's hood. When Tim put the car back in drive, we felt the passenger side drop, and he yelled out, "Oh shit!" The front passenger side of our car dropped into the hollow pit, causing one tire to become lodged as it dangled over the edge. We were stuck. Standing on the side of the road, Tim made a few attempts to get us out, and I called the local fire department for assistance. Tim was embarrassed and concerned that he was blocking traffic.

He politely directed traffic, apologizing to each car squeezing by on the narrow street as we waited for help. Then, a large tour bus pulled around the corner, and I could see the stress in Tim's eyes, realizing the bus would never be able to squeeze through. I stepped in and attempted to prevent the tour bus from coming down our street. Undeterred by my desperate arm waving and hollering, the bus continued driving toward us until forced to stop. I smiled at the driver as he frantically exited the bus, aggressively yelling at us to move our car. I calmly said, "I waved and told you not to come down this road; you should have heeded my warning." Though I was calm, Tim was mortified at the predicament, and I could sense his tension mounting.

Initially, the driver was highly irritated that the bus was trapped, but after realizing the situation was out of our control, he calmed down. Looking for a way to add levity to the tense predicament, I offered the bus driver a different solution. We could either wait for the firetruck to arrive, or he could ask the passengers on his bus for volunteers to lift our car from the hole and unblock the road. Within seconds, a large group of tall, strong Norwegian tourists piled out of the tour bus and lifted the car out of the hole as I looked on.

Taking videos and pictures, I laughed hysterically at the situation unfolding. The tension melted away, and we high-fived our rescuers, offering to buy them all a beer. What started as a misfortune became an unforgettable and happy memory. Soon, we were out of Portugal and arriving in Marrakech.

Once in Marrakech, witnessing Tim's appreciation for the beauty and history we explored and the genuine way he interacted with the local villagers drew me to him. He took nothing for granted and treasured our time together. One experience at a time, I could feel the magnetic pull of our souls connecting. While there, we had the privilege of climbing the Atlas Mountains and visiting the people of a Berber village. We both loved adventure and rode a side-by-side buggy through the dry, dusty heat of the Agafay Desert as the sand painted our skin a new shade of brown. We playfully rode camels and shopped together for gifts in the Medina marketplace, capturing hundreds of photos of our adventures and growing love.

One afternoon, we booked hammam massages. Unsure what to expect, I had heard to set aside inhibitions and keep an open mind. We anxiously walked into the hotel spa holding hands, open to exploring a unique experience. I loved Tim's willingness to jump right in with spontaneity. We were handed the equivalent of a paper loincloth to cover our private parts, then put into a steam room to lie side by side on a warm marble stone. Shortly, a female masseuse moved me into a private room, and a male masseuse took Tim to his room.

In our private rooms, they laid us down on a massive, heated marble slab. After layers of scrubs and mud, they massaged every inch of our bodies, with little left for the imagination. When they were finished massaging, a hose connected to the ceiling was used to vigorously wash off all the layers of mud as the water spilled into the floor drains.

After our experiences, Tim and I sat with hot tea and shared stories of our massages. Completely relaxed, we took a nap and swam in a private pool at our villa before getting ready for an elegant evening dinner event. The trip was beyond anything I could have envisioned; it was romantic and enchanting.

While at dinner events, I met several of Tim's colleagues from his extensive career in the automotive industry. One of the most surprising and refreshing things I learned from them was that Tim never brought a plus-one in all the years he attended the company's worldwide trips. Many were eager to know the first woman he brought on company travels.

A woman I had befriended came and sat beside me at one of the dinners. Her eyes filled with tears, and with delight in her voice, she expressed how pleased she was that I had come into Tim's life. She shared that Tim had attended numerous extravagant company trips without a partner. She and others had a high regard for Tim, not only as a work colleague but as an authentic and kind soul; they had hoped he would find someone to share his life with one day.

Through these conversations, I realized Tim was not only highly respected in his industry, but that his thoughtful disposition sincerely touched the hearts of others. Witnessing his colleagues' admiration and acknowledgment of his character and integrity was reassuring and intensified my attraction to him. Discovering that he could bring a plus- one on all the previous elaborate company travels but chose not to spoke volumes. It reaffirmed his honesty that he wasn't looking for something casual and that all his sentiments about finding true love and building a life together were legitimate and honorable. Tim's actions matched his words, and that far outweighed his taking me on an extravagant trip.

The lavish evening events coupled with adventurous daytime activities were extraordinary, but for me, that trip was more valuable than I imagined. It allowed me to see Tim through numerous lenses, exposing his loving and generous heart. Each layer revealed what I desired to find: another tender soul to love. My heart was full of hope once more.

Following that trip, the beautiful journey of our love story blossomed as we enjoyed quiet nights at home, giggling on the couch, watching movies, spending time with family and friends, and traveling the world. Meeting in our fifties and having whole lives and experiences that shaped us, we came to the table with patterns and routines that we needed to learn to weave together through compromise and compassion.

We were physically attracted to each other from the start, but that was the easy part. We had to weave together our habits and families. Not having kids of his own, Tim took his time while patiently giving Maddie and Jake the space they needed to open up to him. When I first sent the kids a picture of Tim, one of their first comments was, "Mom, homeboy is jacked!" This gave us all a good laugh and was an instant icebreaker. Witnessing their relationships blossom through trust, respect, laughter, and long conversations filled my heart with joy. Slowly, I watched my children's hearts open up to loving Tim, and new bonds were formed as he became an integral part of their lives. With our fair share of different approaches to everyday life, I was surprised that building a life together felt seamless.

Allowing our shared values and love for our families to intertwine organically felt like home. I found it endearing that he maintained a close and loving relationship with his mom, including taking her on her dream vacations. The idea of creating a life with Tim was revitalizing and felt harmonious. He was so excited over the possibilities of our life together that he often expressed his love for me through handwritten poems and songs. I found his gentleness and passion for our relationship refreshing.

The tragic loss of my adoring father came just months after we began dating. Fortunately, he had the opportunity to spend time getting to know Tim. Although my dad had mourned the death of Jeff immensely, he quickly warmed up to Tim. One evening, after leaving my home, my dad pulled his car back into the driveway to make the beautiful gesture of embracing me and Tim with one more large bear hug and express to us that he was happy I had found such a wonderful man to love me once again. I am grateful he took the time to share that moment with us; I will forever cherish it.

Although my heart was ready and open to exploring my newfound love, there was an internal conflict that I was still resolving. I was wrestling with the duality of my love for Jeff, which remained, and my growing love for Tim. *How was it possible for me to love another man as much as I had loved Jeff?* I realized I had experienced a familiar contrasting feeling of love when I was pregnant with Jake. At that time, I had wondered how I could ever love another child as much as I loved Maddie, my first. As a mom of two, I soon discovered that our heart's capacity has no limits if we allow it to expand to its full potential. Remembering how my heart expanded, I recognized why my love for Jeff and Tim could coexist.

My grieving would live with me forever in different measurements, but the pain didn't need to end before I opened and committed my heart once more. I could weave the happiness I was experiencing with

Tim through the grief of the beautiful memories I'd had with Jeff. Tim and Jeff had similarities and differences, but they were still their own individuals. Although it was difficult at first, I made a conscious effort never to compare Tim to Jeff. They each possessed many charming and unique qualities.

When Tim first told me he loved me, he said I didn't need to say it back, only if and when I was ready. My mind negotiated with my heart for weeks until, one day, I freed the words from my tongue and told Tim that I loved him too. I was finally ready to embrace love again fully.

For two years, our love and passion intensified as we continued to weave our lives together at home and travel the world at every possible chance. We spent time exploring the fjord lands of New Zealand, snorkeling in Fiji, golfing in Hawaii, riding horseback along the turquoise waters in Turks and Caicos, driving Vespas through the Tuscany countryside, and witnessing the Pope's mass inside St. Peter's Basilica. It was thrilling to experience a new love in some of the most romantic settings in the world. To find love again while enjoying incredible life experiences together felt like a dream. Tim eventually rented out his place and moved in with me so we could continue to build our life together.

The next chapter of my life unfolded in vivid colors as we embraced our differences and blended our lives. Tim, who loved riding his Harley-Davidson on the weekends, knew I was afraid to be on a motorcycle on the open road. After moving in, he slowly and carefully rode me through the neighborhood, edging out my fears in an effort for us to spend time together doing something he loved. Eventually, we branched out on a few streets nearby until I became more comfortable. He was kind and patient with my apprehension, and before long, I trusted him to take me out onto the highway. We drove his Harley down the Pacific Coast Highway, my arms tightly wrapped around his strong muscular frame, the ocean breeze at our backs, and the road ahead filled with promise.

One of my dating concerns was how my new partner would react to the place I held in my heart for Jeff. From the start, Tim encouraged me to wear the rings Jeff gave me and to continue displaying Jeff's photos and urn. It was a delicate balance of continuing to honor Jeff and being respectful of Tim. While I appreciated his willingness to honor Jeff in our home and on special anniversaries, I also knew I needed to ensure that Tim knew how much I loved him. My heart would always remember Jeff and our love, but there was still plenty of room to build loving memories with Tim. He created a beautiful and safe place for me to talk about and honor Jeff freely.

Early on in our relationship, I shared with Tim that one day, I wanted to write a memoir about me and Jeff and the journey we'd experienced together. I knew it would take an incredibly confident and unique man to accept that Jeff would always be woven into the fabric of my heart. Tim supported my decision and encouraged me to take on the newest hat I would wear: author. I bounced book ideas and concepts off him and spent countless late-night hours after work and on the weekends writing. Tim thoughtfully made dinner and brought me wine while I sat in my dimly lit, candle-filled room, working on the book about me and Jeff.

While he fully supported my book writing, I was acutely aware that it would likely be a challenging read for him. I gave Tim a guilt-free, judgment-free pass, never to read the book if he chose. If the roles were reversed, I'm not sure I would want to hear the details of how madly in love Tim was before he met me. We had talked extensively about Jeff's cancer journey and all the painful details of my life before him, including what that last day was like. Tim didn't need to read the book to support me. He had shown his support in countless ways, which were meaningful to me, from helping me work through challenging chapter ideas to popping champagne as I completed the final chapter.

For three and a half years, Jeff and I had learned to live while he was dying. We taught ourselves to appreciate the beauty in the ordinary and find gratitude in moments of darkness. Moving forward, it became crucial for me to continue living in that manner, to appreciate and grab hold of life's opportunities. Little did I know how essential that would be for what lay around the corner.

After two years of dating, Tim and I created a new life together and shared the most intimate parts of our hearts. It was then that Tim's company offered him a position as the Chief Sales Officer for Australia. My immediate reaction was to embrace it fully without hesitation. With the profound firsthand knowledge that life is precious, I knew I couldn't let an exciting opportunity to move across the world with Tim be overwhelmed by fear of the unknown. It was a once-in-a-lifetime opportunity that few are presented with, so together, Tim and I decided to jump in and let faith guide us.

We told our families about the opportunity, and although we all could feel our heartstrings tug thinking about the distance, everyone selflessly supported the move. Tim's company flew us out for an initial trip to Australia to see if moving to Melbourne would fit our lifestyle, and we quickly fell in love with the captivating city down under. We had a couple of months to figure out the logistics of selling my business and packing up our lives to move to the other side of the world. As we embraced the two- year opportunity, we found incredible joy in building a life together in our new city. We saw the experience as a chance to strengthen our relationship while exploring another part of the world in Oceania.

Trepidation and apprehension weighed on my mind as we made the life-changing decision. Two years into our new relationship, Tim and I were still learning about each other. Even so, one thing was certain: We were both fully committed and wholly in love. Having lived in Southern California for fifty-six years, I needed to find the courage to leave the only life I'd known.

As we packed our memories to move across the world, my heart was overwhelmed and full of so many mixed emotions— elation, heartache, excitement, anxiety, and fear—that I could barely breathe them all in. But overriding them all was my love for Tim and joy for the life-changing opportunity we'd been given. Together, we embraced the leap of faith even though our hearts struggled. The duality of emotions that came with moving halfway around the world forced us far outside our comfort zones. Once again, I couldn't let fear fuel my decision, so I embraced the extraordinary adventure ahead with Tim steadfastly by my side.

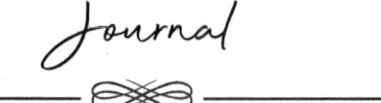

Stepping into a new chapter of life often means holding joy in one hand and grief in the other. Reflect on a time when you embraced something new, whether a relationship, opportunity, or adventure, while still carrying the love and memories of what came before. How did you let both coexist without diminishing either?

Epilogue

During the first few months of our new journey, I put the final touches on my book in my new office in our high-rise city apartment in Melbourne, as Tim and I lived our grand adventure in Australia. With a whole new city lifestyle, filled with abundant wildlife and natural beauty to explore, we continued to discover more about each other, loving every minute of our new life and exquisite love. I was so grateful for all God had given me. I often reflected on the beauty of the new life I was living and the terror of many days that now lay in the past.

I was asked countless times how I stayed optimistic and faithful to God during those unimaginable days of facing death after Jeff's diagnosis. People wondered how I never let go of hope and joy while facing the fear of losing the love of my life every day for so many years. There was a time when I didn't have an answer, but now I do.

One of the mantras my mind has set on default is that no matter the challenge we're facing, most things in life are temporary; they will pass. Remember that the obstacles in our path are a space for growth, and if we take the time to pause amid heartbreak, no matter how critical the situation may be, there is always beauty to be discovered. Keeping my eyes and heart open and finding gratitude in seemingly insurmountable moments was vital to my substance and survival.

Leaning into my faith and carving out time to reflect, recharge, and replenish my energy and soul allowed me to find my breath during life's turbulent moments, creating beauty amidst sorrow. We can't avoid tough conversations, because how we say goodbye to our loved ones can change the trajectory of how we weave happiness through grief.

In this marathon of life, I don't want to look back one day with significant regrets, pondering *What if?* and *If only I had.*

We miss 100 percent of the shots we never take.

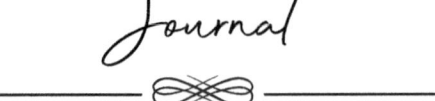

Life's hardest seasons often hold unexpected beauty if we're willing to look for it. Think about a challenge you've faced that, in time, revealed moments of grace, growth, or gratitude. What helped you keep your heart open enough to find light in the darkness?

I would love to stay connected. You can reach me at: stephanie@thestephanieduran.com

Visit me online:

Follow me on Instagram:

www.ingramcontent.com/pod-product-compliance
Lightning Source LLC
LaVergne TN
LVHW061540070526
838199LV00077B/6857